# THERAPEUTIC KEY;

OR,

# PRACTICAL GUIDE

FOR THE

# HOMŒOPATHIC TREATMENT

OF

# ACUTE DISEASES.


BY

I. D. JOHNSON, M. D.


*Similia similibus curantur.*


PHILADELPHIA:
F. E. BOERICKE, No. 635 ARCH STREET.
*NEW YORK:* BOERICKE & TAFEL, 145 GRAND ST.
1872.

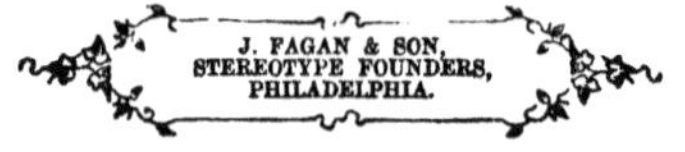
J. FAGAN & SON,
STEREOTYPE FOUNDERS,
PHILADELPHIA.

# PREFACE.

THIS little volume is simply what its title indicates, a "Practical Guide" to aid the memory of the practitioner at the bed-side.

The necessity for a work like this must be apparent to every Homœopathic physician, even of limited experience. The fact that many of our distinguished practitioners carry with them, in their daily rounds of practice, the larger works to refer to, clearly indicates the necessity that exists for a book of this kind. Therefore, it is to supply this deficiency that I now offer this little volume to the Profession, as the fruit of my humble effort. It has been written at irregular and interrupted intervals, amid the pressure of other cares, and is the result of many years' experience, observation, and study. In its preparation I have consulted the best recent and ancient authorities in our English and American Homœopathic literature, and have carefully selected from their rich treasury most of the material it contains. I have given only such symptoms and indications for the exhibition of remedies as have withstood the practical test of experience. Most of these symptoms have been expressly set forth as *characteristics*, or *key-notes*, by Professors Guernsey, Herring, Lippe, Raue, and others, who regard them as preëminently requisite in determining the choice of the remedy. For this reason I have marked these characteristic symptoms with a star (*), to denote their distinctive value. It is not intended, however, that they should determine the choice of the remedy to the exclusion of others, as every symptom possesses a relative value which must correspond with those of the individual case. The symptoms marked in *italics* are likewise characteristic of the remedies, but in a less or subordinate degree.

With respect to the remedies themselves, they have been arranged under the head of each particular disease, in alphabetical order, and many new ones have been added, which will be found to disclose important symptoms not met with elsewhere.

The diseases have likewise been arranged in alphabetical order in the body of the work, as well as in the Contents, and can therefore be consulted with the greatest facility.

For convenience, it is desirable that a book of this kind should be made to occupy as little space as possible, and for this reason I have considered only acute diseases, or that class requiring prompt treatment, and which does not admit of time to consult larger works at the office. A chapter, however, has been devoted to the treatment of "Poisoning," and also one on "Apparent Death from Drowning," "Suffocation," &c., which will be found of great practical importance to the junior, as well as to the older members of the Profession.

In conclusion, I may say that it has been my earnest endeavor to make this little volume one of practical utility. How far I have succeeded in the execution of this design, I leave to the just decision of those who are qualified to judge.

I. D. JOHNSON.

KENNETT SQUARE, Pa.,
July, 1871.

# CONTENTS.

# PRACTICAL GUIDE

## IN THE TREATMENT OF

# ACUTE DISEASES.

---

### ABSCESS.

**Therapeutics.** Special indications.

**Acon.** The tumor is swollen, red, and shining. Violent cutting pains; the parts burn, as from hot coals. Great nervous and vascular excitement. * Gets desperate about the pain, and declares that something *must be done.* * Great fear and anxiety of mind. Aggravation in the evening, and during the night.

**Ars.** The abscess threatens to become gangrenous, and is accompanied with *great debility.* * Violent burning pains; the parts burn like fire. Restless tossing about. * Great thirst, but can drink but little. Aggravation during rest, and better by motion.

**Asafœtida.** The abscess discharges a thin, fetid pus; is very painful to contact, especially the surrounding parts. * Pains, with numbness of the affected parts. Nervous, hysterical, scrofulous individuals.

**Bell.** The tumor is much swollen, hard, and of an erysipelatous appearance. Pressing, burning, stinging or throbbing pains. * Pains which appear suddenly and leave as suddenly. * The parts have a hot, dry sensation, with much throbbing; they get worse about 3 P. M. Mammary abscesses.

**Bryonia.** Mostly in the beginning, when the abscess is hard, swollen, and *feels heavy.* The tumor alternates in color, and is either very red or very pale. * Stitching pains, aggravated by the slightest motion. * Hard, dry stools, as if burnt.

**Hepar.** * Where suppuration is inevitable. Throbbing pains, frequently preceded by a chill. Scrofulous persons, and after the abuse of mercury.

**Ledum.** In the early stage, when the abscess is distended and hard. * Stinging and tearing pains, aggravated by heat. *Tensive, hard swelling*, with tearing pains.

**Mezer.** Abscesses that occur in fibrous and tendinous structures, or where they arise from the abuse of mercury. Stinging and throbbing pains, worse at night and from contact or motion.

**Puls.** The abscess bleeds easily, with stinging or cutting pains. Violent itching, burning, and stinging in the periphery of the abscess. Pus copious and yellow. After violent and long continued inflammations. * Mild, tearful persons; they weep at everything, be it good or bad.

**Rhus tox.** Especially for abscesses of the axillary or parotid glands. Stinging and gnawing pains in the tumor, which is very painful to touch. Discharge of a bloody-serous matter. * Pain worse during rest, and relieved by moving the affected parts.

**Silicea** Where suppuration is imminent, or in cases where the discharge becomes fetid, thin, and watery. Several fistulous openings form, which are very slow to heal. * In whitlow, where the pain is intense and the swelling unabated.

**Sulph.** Inveterate cases, when there is a profuse discharge of matter, with emaciation, hectic fever, &c. Where there is a constant tendency to a return of the disease. Scrofulous persons who are frequently troubled with boils. * Psoric diathesis. * Lean persons who walk stooping.

---

## AFTER-PAINS.

**Therapeutics.** Special indications.

**Arnica.** Sore feeling all through the patient as if from a bruise. The pains are not very violent, but there is a bruised sore feeling, with pressure on the bladder and retention of urine.

**Bell.** * Severe bearing-down pains, as if all would be forced through the external organs. * The pains come on suddenly, and leave just as suddenly. Fulness and great tenderness of the abdomen. Sleepiness, but cannot sleep.

**Bryonia.** * The pains are of a stitch-like character, and are excited by the least motion. The patient is exceedingly irritable.

**Cham.** Great nervous excitement, with restless tossing about. The *pains are very distressing,* and she becomes almost furious. * Very impatient, can hardly answer one civilly. Dark lochial discharge.

**Coff.** Great sensitiveness, with general excitability. * Violent pains, driving her almost to despair. Extreme wakefulness.

**Cup. acet.** * Terrible cramping pains, often accompanied with cramps in the extremities. Spasms, with nausea and vomiting.

**Ignatia.** The pains are cramp-like and pressing, resembling labor pains. * Sadness and sighing, with an empty feeling at the pit of the stomach.

**Nux vom.** When the pains are aching and more like colic. Violent contractive pains in the uterus. * Every pain causes an inclination to go to stool. Much pain in the small of the back, worse by turning in bed.

**Puls.** Severe colicky pains extending to the back. The pains grow worse towards evening. Bad taste in the mouth, with desire to vomit. * Persons of a mild, tearful disposition. Thirstlessness.

**Secale cor.** Excessive uterine contractions, which are long continued. * In thin, feeble, scrawny females, or women who have borne many children. Thin, offensive lochial discharge.

**Sulph.** Flashes of heat, and frequent weak, faint spells. Feet either cold or burning hot, particularly in the soles. * Constant heat in the top of the head.

**Sulph. acid.** Great sense of general weakness. * A sense of trembling all over, without absolute trembling. Profuse perspiration, with great debility.

## AMENORRHŒA.

**Therapeutics.** Special indications.

**Aconite.** If the suppression is the result of direct application of cold. Congestion of blood to the head or chest, with flushed face. Shooting and beating pains in the head, with delirium or stupefaction. * Vertigo with faintness on rising from a recumbent position.

**Arsen.** Pale waxen color of the face. Great prostration of strength from the least exertion. Loss of appetite; sadness and melancholy. Fear of death and of being left alone. Much chilliness: wants more clothes on, or to be near the fire. * Intense thirst, but drinks little. * Sufferings all worse after midnight.

**Bell.** Throbbing headache at the approach of each menstrual period. Red face, with determination of blood to the head when stooping. * Bearing-down pain in the hypogastrium as if the menses would appear. * She cannot bear light or noise.

**Bryonia.** Swimming in the head, with painful pressure in the temples. *Bleeding of the nose,* and bursting headache. Drawing pains in the lower part of the abdomen. * Hard, dry stools as if burnt. * Symptoms all worse by the least motion.

**Calc. carb.** Scrofulous, rickety subjects. The menstrual period is preceded by swelling and soreness of the breasts, headache, colic, shiverings, and leucorrhœa. * Cold, damp feet, and swelling at the pit of the stomach. * Dizziness on going up-stairs.

**Causticum.** Yellow, discolored complexion. Weakly, scrofulous subjects with glandular swellings. Melancholy mood; she looks on the dark side of everything. Hysterical spasms and pinching pain in the sacrum. Leucorrhœa particularly at night.

**Cham.** Pressure towards the genital organs, like labor-pains. Cutting colic, and drawing in the thighs previous to a menstrual period. * She is very irritable, can hardly answer one civilly. * One cheek red and the other pale. Passing of large quantities of colorless urine.

**China.** Pale, sickly complexion. Weakness of digestion; fulness and distention of the abdomen, particularly after eating. * Debility from loss of animal fluids.

**Cocculus.** Leucorrhœa in place of the menses. * During the menstrual period, she is extremely weak. Sometimes a few drops of black blood are discharged. Nervous hysterical subjects.

**Coloc.** Amenorrhœa from anger and silent grief. * Severe colicky pains which compel one to bend double. Great anguish and restlessness.

**Conium.** Much vertigo, particularly when lying down, or when turning over in bed. * At every menstrual effort, the breasts enlarge, become sore and painful. Much difficulty in voiding urine; it intermits in its flow.

**Crocus.** Sensation as if the menses would appear, with colic and dragging down in the direction of the pudendum. * Sensation of something moving in the abdomen. Discharge of thick, black, stringy blood from the nose.

**Dulc.** Amenorrhœa from exposure to cold, or from getting wet. * At each menstrual period a rash shows itself upon the skin. Every time she takes cold has urticaria or some other eruption on the skin.

**Graph.** Suppression of the menses, with a sense of weight in the arms and lower extremities An occasional show of the menses, the discharge being very pale and scant. Swelling and coldness of the feet. * Eruptions on the skin oozing out a sticky fluid.

**Kali carb.** Amenorrhœa, with anasarca and ascites. Pains in the abdomen resembling false laborpains. Shortness of breath and violent palpitation of the heart * Little sac-like swelling over the upper eyelid, in the morning.

**Lyco.** Chronic suppression of the menses; also from fright. *Sour eructations, with nausea and vomiting,* especially in the morning. *Great fulness in the stomach and bowels.* * Red, sandy sediment in the urine.

**Nux mos.** Suppression of the menses from exposure to wet, with severe pains in the abdomen. * Irregular menstruation, blood thick and dark.

*Sleepiness and inclination to faint.* * Great dryness of the tongue, particularly after sleeping. Pain in the back as if broken and bruised. Enormous distention of the abdomen after eating.

**Pulsatilla.** Suppression, especially from *getting the feet wet.* Aching pains over the forehead, with pressure on the vertex. Vertigo, with buzzing in the ears. Stitching toothache, the pains suddenly shift from one side to the other. Palpitation of the heart Pain in the stomach, with nausea and vomiting. * Constant chilliness even in a warm room. * Persons of a mild tearful disposition, with a tendency to sadness. Symptoms all worse in the evening.

**Sepia.** Frequent paroxysms of hysteric or nervous headache. Toothache, with great sensitiveness of the dental nerves. * Sallow complexion or dingy spots on the face. Nervous debility and great disposition to sweat. * Painful sensation of emptiness at the pit of the stomach.

**Sulphur.** Aching and tensive pain in the head, especially from the occiput to the neck. Rush of blood to the head, with a whizzing noise in the brain. * Constant heat in the top of the head. Pale, sickly complexion, blue margins around the eyes. Frequent weak, faint spells through the day. * She gets very hungry about 11 A. M., cannot wait for her dinner. Great nervous debility, especially in the lower extremities.

**Verat. alb.** Nervous headache at every menstrual period, with hysterical symptoms. Pale, livid face, and cold sweat upon the forehead. Cold hands, feet, and nose. * Great weakness, with frequent spells of fainting.

---

## APHTHÆ.

**Therapeutics.** Special indications.

**Aconite.** Dry, hot skin, with much heat about the head. Constant restlessness, cries much, bites its fist, and has a green, watery diarrhœa. * Excessive sensibility to the least touch.

**Arsen.** The mouth is reddish-blue, and inflamed. Fetid smell from the mouth; great restlessness. * Green, watery diarrhœa, attended with great weakness.

**Borax.** Red blisters on the tongue, as if the skin were pulled off. Shrivelling up of the mucous membrane. The child cries when taking the breast as if in pain. Light yellow slimy stools. * Fear of falling from a downward motion.

**Calc. c.** Scrofulous children, especially during dentition. * Large, open fontanelles. Hard, undigested stools of a light color. * Cold, damp feet.

**Cham.** Child starts and jumps much during sleep. Wants different things, and rejects them when presented. * Very uneasy, and must be carried all the time.

**Mercurius.** Tongue inflamed, swollen, and ulcerated on the edges. The gums bleed, and incline to ulcerate about the teeth. Very fetid breath. * Profuse secretion of saliva in the mouth. Dysenteric diarrhœa, with griping and tenesmus.

**Nitric ac.** Mouth full of fetid ulcers, with putrid smelling breath. * Ptyalism of a corrosive nature, causing fresh ulcers to break out on the lips, chin, or cheeks. Bleeding of the gums. Particularly if there should be a syphilitic discrasia.

**Nux vom.** If the disease assumes the character of stomatitis. Painful swelling of the gums, with burning or beating pains. Fetid ulcers or blisters in the mouth, on the gums, palate, or tongue. * Constipation, with frequent urging to stool. Irritable mood.

**Staph.** Spongy excrescence on the gums and in the mouth. Vesicles under the tongue. Mouth and tongue ulcerated and covered with blisters. Sickly complexion, with sunken cheeks, hollow eyes surrounded with blue margins. * The aphthous patches seem to bleed easily, and the gums are spongy.

**Sulphur.** Thick whitish or brownish aphthous coating on the tongue. Blisters and aphthæ in the mouth, with burning and soreness, especially when eating. Ptyalism or bloody saliva. *Acrid, slimy or*

2

*greenish diarrhœa excoriating the parts.* * The child does not take its usual long nap, but wakens often.

**Sulph. ac.** The mouth appears very painful, and the child is very weak. Vesicles on the inner side of the cheeks; ulcers on the gums. Profuse flow of tasteless saliva. * Diarrhœa with great debility, and inclination to sweat.

---

## APOPLEXIA.

**Therapeutics.** Special indications.

**Aconite.** Congestion of blood to the head, with heat and redness of the face. Eyes red, sparkling, and prominent, with dilated pupils; fixed look. Paralysis of the tongue, with trembling, stammering speech. *Great difficulty in swallowing.* Pulse full and hard, but not intermittent.

**Arnica.** Head hot, while the rest of the body is cool. Paralysis of the limbs, especially the left side. Loss of consciousness, with stupefaction and stertorous breathing. Staring eyes and contraction of the pupils. * Sighing, muttering, and involuntary discharge of fæces and urine.

**Baryta c.** Apoplexy of aged persons, and those of intemperate habits. Paralysis of the limbs (right side). *Disturbed consciousness, with childish gesticulations* and inability to keep the body erect.

**Belladon.** Face swollen, bluish, and dark-red. Distention of the veins of the head and neck * Visible throbbing of the carotid and temporal arteries. Drowsiness with loss of consciousness and of speech. Paralysis of the limbs, especially of the right side. * Mouth drawn to one side; difficult or impossible deglutition. * Loss of sight, smell, and speech. Involuntary emissions of urine.

**Cocc.** The paroxysm is preceded by a *stupid feeling in the head, and vertigo.* Convulsive motions of the eyes. Paralysis, especially of the *lower limbs*, with insensibility. * Head and face hot, feet cold.

**Hyos.** * Sudden falling down with a shriek.

Loss of consciousness and of speech; foam at the mouth. Constriction of the throat, and inability to swallow. Brown-red, swollen face, and staring distorted eyes, with dilatation of the pupils. Paralysis of the bladder and sphincter ani. * Twitching and jerking of all the muscles in the body.

**Lachesis.** Apoplexia with paralysis of the left side, and coldness of the hands as if dead. *Mouth drawn to one side, mostly to the left.* Attack preceded by frequent absence of mind or vertigo. * Cannot bear anything to touch his neck. Entire inability to swallow.

**Nux vom.** The paroxysm is preceded by vertigo with headache and buzzing in the ears, or nausea with urging to vomit. Swelling and redness of the face. Stupefaction, with stertorous breathing. * Paralysis of the lower jaw, and often the lower extremities, which are cold and without sensation. Habitual constipation. Persons of sedentary habits, who live upon highly seasoned food and stimulating drinks.

**Opium.** * The patient lies in a state of sopor and unconsciousness, with half open eyes and dilated pupils. Redness, bloatedness, and heat of the face. * Respiration labored, snoring and rattling. *Convulsive motions of the extremities, or tetanic stiffness of the whole body.* Slow pulse.

**Hydroc. ac** The features are spasmodically distorted, the eyes fixed and turned upwards. Pupils immovable; breathing stertorous, and pulse almost imperceptible. * Paralysis of the œsophagus; fluids pass down into the stomach with a gurgling sound.

**Laurocerasus.** Sudden attack of apoplexia where the patient falls down without any precursory symptoms. Eyes staring, or lightly closed; *pupils dilated,* or contracted and immovable. Slow, feeble, moaning, or rattling breathing.

**Pulsatilla.** Stupefaction and loss of consciousness. Bloated and bluish-red face. Loss of motion, violent palpitation of the heart, and almost complete suppression of the pulse. Restless sleep and tossing about. * Persons of a mild tearful disposition.

## APPARENT DEATH.

**Treatment.** In asphyxia from **Cold**, always place the body in a *cold* room, and cover it with snow, or bathe it in ice-cold water until the limbs become soft and flexible, then place it in a dry bed and rub briskly with flannel, at the same time try to induce artificial respiration by Dr. Hall's method, explained under the head of "Asphyxia from Drowning." As soon as there are signs of returning life, give small injections of *coffee* without milk, and if the patient can swallow, give him spoonful doses of *coffee* to drink.

For the severe burning pains which usually follow resuscitation from intense cold: **Acon.**, **Ars.**, **Carb. veg.**, or **Bryo.**, will be found sufficient.

Asphyxia from **Drowning**: "Place the body in a horizontal position, *face down*, with one wrist under the forehead. Now, with one hand upon the back and the other upon the abdomen, press gently for about two seconds, then turn the body well upon its side, and after a couple of seconds place it again upon the face and repeat the pressing as before; in this way strive to induce artificial respiration by the alternate pressure upon the abdomen and rotation of the body." Meantime have the limbs rubbed briskly upward, and the wet articles of clothing replaced by dry warm ones from the bystanders.

In addition to the mechanical means resorted to, a dose of **Lachesis** may be placed upon the tongue, or administered as an injection. **Tartar em.** is also a valuable remedy in these cases.

Asphyxia from **Hanging**, **Choking**, &c. Endeavor to induce artificial respiration by the same method as recommended for drowning, and give **Opium** or **Tartar em.** by injection.

Asphyxia from **Lightning**. Place the patient immediately in a freshly made opening in the ground, in a half sitting posture, with his face toward the sun, and cover him all over with fresh earth. Give **Nux vom.** as soon as there are any signs of returning life.

Asphyxia from **Carbonic-acid Gas**. Bathe the

patient with *vinegar*, and let him inhale the vapor; apply cold water to the head and warmth to the feet. If there is congestion to the head, loss of consciousness, throbbing of the carotids, and red, bloated face, give **Belladonna.** If the face is purplish and swollen, with soporous sleep, stertorous breathing, and vomiting, give **Opium.** If the patient is very much excited, talks much and rapidly, complains of shooting pains, or if it seems to him as if he were flying, feels giddy when lying down, give **Coffea.**

---

## ARTHRITIS.

**Therapeutics.** Special indications.

**Aconite.** Synochal fever. The parts affected are swollen, red, and shining. Tearing or stitching pains, less when moving the parts. * The pains are intolerable at night, the patient becoming desperate. Aggravation from the use of wine or other stimulants.

**Arnica.** Hard, red swelling of the joints, particularly of the knee. Violent pains as if sprained or contused, with a sensation as if *resting upon something hard.* * Great fear of being struck by persons coming near him. Aggravation by moving the parts.

**Arsen.** Swelling of the feet, hot, shining, with burning red spots. * Burning pains — the parts burn like fire. Wants to be in a warm room. Great anguish, restlessness, and fear of death. Intense thirst, but drinks little. Symptoms all worse at night, particularly after midnight.

**Bell.** Wide-spreading redness and swelling of the parts, like erysipelas. * Stitching, burning, and throbbing pains, which come on suddenly and leave as suddenly. Throbbing headache. * Sleepiness, but cannot sleep. Symptoms all worse at 3 P. M.

**Bryonia.** Red or pale tensive swelling, particularly of the joints. * Stitching, tearing pains, aggravated by motion and relieved by rest. * Patient wants to remain perfectly quiet. Extremely irritable;

everything makes him angry * Dry, hard stools, as if burnt.

**Colch.** Little or no swelling of the affected part; the skin is rose-colored, and leaves a white spot under the pressure of the finger. * Paroxysms of tearing, stitching, jerking pains, particularly in the finger-joints. * Urine dark and scanty, depositing a whitish sediment. Pains intolerable at night.

**Ferrum acet.** The patient has a pale, consumptive look. Several joints are affected at the same time; the pains are violent, stinging, and tearing, obliging him to move the parts constantly. * The least emotion or pain produces a red, flushed face.

**Mercurius.** Red and hot swelling of the affected joints. The pains are drawing and lacerating, or the joints feel as if dislocated; *worse in cold damp weather*, and at night. * Much perspiration, which affords no relief.

**Nux vom.** The pains are tensive, *jerking*, or pulling, worse in the morning, from mental exertion, from motion and slight contact; *but strong pressure relieves.* * Persons of intemperate or sedentary habits, and those who live on rich and highly-seasoned food. Constipation, or morning diarrhœa.

**Phosphorus.** Arthritic affections of the wrist and finger-joints. Pains as if lacerated or sprained, worse early in the morning or in the evening. * Long, narrow, hard stools, very difficult to expel. * Sensation of weakness and emptiness in the abdomen. Lean, slender persons.

**Puls.** Red and hot swelling of the parts affected, particularly of the knee-joints and feet. The pains are tearing, stitching, burning. * Erratic pains, shifting rapidly from one joint to another. Aggravation *towards evening*, or at night. * Craves fresh cool air; worse in a warm room. * Persons of a mild, tearful disposition.

**Rhus tox.** Rheumatic gout; the joints are red, shining, and swollen. Stiffness and lameness of the affected parts. The pains are tearing, burning, or as if sprained. * Aggravation on first moving the limb after rest, or *during rest; relieved by motion.*

**Sabina**. Swelling, redness, and stitches in the big toe. Nodosities of the joints. Pains tearing and stinging, almost insupportable when the limbs hang down; *relief in the open air*

---

## ASTHMA.

**Therapeutics**. Special indications.

**Aconite**. Shortness of breath, especially when sleeping. Paroxysms of suffocation, with anxiety and restlessness. Dyspnœa, with inability to take a deep breath. Spasmodic, rough, croaking cough, with constriction of the windpipe. *Great fear and anxiety of mind, with nervous excitability. *Fear of death, predicts the day he will die.

**Arsenicum**. Anxious and oppressed shortness of breath, with labored breathing, particularly when ascending an eminence. Attacks of *suffocation, especially at night*, or in the evening in bed, with wheezing respiration. *Great anguish, extreme restlessness, and fear of death. *Extreme thirst, and drinks but little. *Cannot lie down for fear of suffocation. Wants to be in a warm room.

**Belladonna**. Paroxysm mostly in the afternoon or evening. *Sensation as if dust were in the lungs, better when bending the head back, and when holding the breath. Face and eyes red, and head hot. Dry, spasmodic cough, especially at night. Uneasiness and beating in the chest. *Sleepiness, but cannot sleep. Plethoric individuals and young people.

**Bryonia**. Increased difficulty of breathing when talking, and during any kind of exercise. *Patient wants to remain perfectly quiet, as the least exertion makes him worse. Frequent dry cough, or cough with expectoration of a quantity of mucus. Stitches in the chest, especially during an inspiration or when coughing. *Sitting up in bed causes nausea and fainting. *Dry, hard stools, as if burnt.

**Cham**. Oppression in the chest, as if from incarcerated flatulence in the epigastrium. Constriction of the upper part of the chest, with soreness when coughing. Hoarseness and cough from rattling of mucus in the trachea. * Much hot perspiration about the face and head. One cheek red and the other pale. * Is very impatient, can hardly answer one civilly. Especially adapted to children; they are very cross, and *want to be carried all the time.*

**China.** Suffocative fits, as from mucus in the larynx, in the evening in bed. Difficult inspiration and quick expiration. * The patient appears as if dying. Cough, with difficult expectoration of clear, tenacious mucus. Worse at night and after drinking. * Better every other day.

**Conium.** Asthma, particularly in the morning on waking. Rattling in the chest. Dry, tickling cough, increasing when lying down, with oppression of the chest. * Face of a bluish-red color. Pale urine, voided with difficulty. Attacks mostly in wet weather.

**Ferrum.** Asthma most violent when lying down, obliging one to sit up. Spasmodic cough with expectoration of transparent, tenacious mucus. * With every paroxysm or fit of coughing, the face becomes fiery-red. Always better when walking slowly about.

**Ipecac.** Spasmodic asthma, with violent *contraction in the throat and chest.* Contraction of the chest with short and panting breathing. * Rattling noise in the bronchial tubes, during an inspiration. * Suffocation threatens from constriction in the throat and chest; worse from the least motion. * Nausea with a feeling of emptiness about the stomach.

**Kali carb.** Difficult wheezing respiration. Spasmodic asthma, worse about 3 A. M., relieved by sitting up and bending forward, resting the head on the knees. Cough, excited by a tickling in the throat, with sourish expectoration, or of blood-streaked mucus. * Great aversion to being alone.

**Lobelia in.** The attack is preceded or accompanied by a kind of prickly sensation through the whole system, even to the ends of the fingers and toes. Short anxious wheezing respiration. * Sensation as of a foreign body in the throat, impeding breathing and deglutition. Nausea and vomiting with a sense of great emptiness in the stomach.

**Lachesis.** Shortness of breath, after every exertion. Tightness of breathing, with anguish in the chest and great inclination to vomit. * Can bear nothing to touch the larynx, seems as though it would suffocate him. * Aggravation after sleeping, and during rest.

**Phos.** Loud and panting respiration. Spasmodic constriction of the chest. Fatiguing cough, with expectoration of tenacious mucus. * Complete loss of voice. * Sensation of weakness and emptiness in the abdomen. * Long, narrow, hard stools, very difficult to expel. Tall, slender people.

**Sambucus.** Violent dyspnœa, with anguish and danger of suffocation, especially when lying down. * Nightly suffocative paroxysms, with spasmodic constriction of the chest. Mucus rattling in the chest. Especially adapted to children.

**Spongia.** Difficult respiration as if the throat were closed by a plug. Wheezing respiration or slow and deep breathing, as if from debility. * Awakens often in a frigh and feels as if she was suffocating. Hoarse, hollow wheezing cough.

**Silphium lac.** Acute or chronic asthma, with much difficulty of breathing. Wheezing in the chest during an inspiration. Moist cough with copious expectoration of white frothy mucus. Especially in old people.

**Sulphur.** The attack comes on during sleep or in the evening, with a feeling of tightness across the chest, and a sensation as of dust in the air-passages. Dry cough with hoarseness, or *loose cough* with soreness and pressure in the chest. * Frequent weak, faint spells. * Constant heat on top of the head. If the attack was caused by breathing a smoky atmosphere.

**Tartar em.** Anxious oppression, difficulty of breathing and shortness of breath, with desire to sit erect. * When the patient coughs, it seems as if the bronchial tubes were full of phlegm, but none comes up. Suffocative fits, especially in the evening or in the morning in bed.

**Verat. alb.** The attack mostly occurs in cold, damp weather, and early in the morning. Anguish, suffocation, and oppression about the heart. Coldness of the nose, ears, and lower extremities. * Cold sweat upon the forehead, with great prostration. Exhausting diarrhœa.

---

## ATROPHY OF CHILDREN.

**Therapeutics.** Special indications.

**Æthusa c.** The child throws up its milk soon after nursing, *with great force, suddenly*—then falls asleep as if from exhaustion, to awaken for a fresh supply.

**Arsen.** General emaciation, with dry parchment-like skin. Pale and œdematous swelling of the face. Sunken eyes with blue margins. * Feverish heat, with desire to drink often, but little at a time. Great restlessness and tossing about, particularly at night. Painful, offensive undigested stools. *Prostration* and coldness of the extremities.

**Baryta c.** Swelling and induration of the glands. Emaciation, bloated face, swollen abdomen and constant desire to sleep. Indisposed to work or play. * Scrofulous children that do not grow.

**Bell.** Glandular swellings, painful or suppurating. Eyelids inflamed and ulcers on the cornea. * Child sleepy, but cannot get to sleep. * Sudden starting and jumping during sleep. Children with premature intellects.

**Bryo. alb.** The child throws up its food immediately after taking it. Mouth and lips very dry, with thirst for large quantities of water. * Child is very irritable and wants to be very quiet. * Dry, hard stools, as if burnt.

**Calc. c.** Large *head with open fontanelles.* Dry and flabby skin. Enlargement and hardness of the abdomen. * General emaciation with a good appetite. Debility and weakness after the least exercise. Diarrhœa, with clay-colored stools. * Cold, damp feet. * Much perspiration about the head. Cough with rattling of mucus in the bronchia.

**China.** Pale, sickly appearance of the face. Enlargement of the liver and spleen. Copious sweats, especially at night; great debility and prostration. * Painless, undigested, offensive stools. * Abdomen distended with flatulence.

**Mercurius.** Yellow earthy color of the face. Large head and open fontanelles. Swelling and suppuration of the glands. * Slimy or bloody stools, with much straining. * Profuse night sweats. Child is never so well during wet weather.

**Nux vom.** Swelling and hardness of the liver. *Obstinate constipation*, or alternate constipation and diarrhœa. Hunger with aversion to food. Frequent vomiting of the ingesta. Constant desire to lie down. * Cannot sleep after three or four in the morning.

**Phos.** Pale and bloated face. Sunken eyes, with blue circles under the same. Dry, hacking cough. Diarrhœa, with white, watery, undigested stools. Great debility and oppression after the least exercise. * Children of tall, slender stature.

**Puls.** The child seems to be very changeable; gets better for a time, and then without any apparent cause gets worse. * Diarrhœa, especially at night, no two stools alike, so changeable. * Worse towards evening; *better in the open air.*

**Rhus tox.** Herpetic eruptions on the face. Swelling and induration of the glands. Diarrhœa, with thin red mucous stools. * The child always gets worse after twelve o'clock at night.

**Staph.** Hollow eyes, with weary look. Swelling of the submaxillary and cervical glands. Unhealthy, readily ulcerating skin. * Canine hunger, even when the stomach is full of food.

**Sulphur.** The child frequently awakens from sleep with screams. Great voracity, wants to put everything it sees in the mouth. * Diarrhœa, excoriating the anus. * Copious morning sweats, after waking.

## BRONCHITIS.

**Therapeutics.** Special indications.

**Aconite.** Mostly in the commencement of acute attacks. Chill and cynochal fever, dry hot skin, and great restlessness. Short dry cough, with constant irritation in the larynx. * Great fear and anxiety of mind, with nervous excitability. After exposure to dry cold winds.

**Apis mal.** Sensation of soreness in the chest as from a bruise. * Cough, particularly after lying down and sleeping. A clear, tough, stringy phlegm arises in the throat, which causes him to hawk frequently.

**Arsen. alb.** Dry hacking cough, with soreness in the chest as if raw, or moist cough with difficult expectoration consisting of blood-streaked mucus. Oppression and difficulty of breathing, obliging him to sit up. * Great thirst, but drinks little. Restlessness, debility, and fear of death.

**Bellad.** Congestion of blood to the head, with visible pulsation of the carotids. Face flushed and eyes red. * Great fulness in the head, or pains as if it would split. Hot skin, with inclination to perspire. Spasmodic cough which does not allow one time to breathe. Children cry after every coughing spell on account of the pain. Sleepy, but cannot sleep. * Starting and jumping during sleep.

**Bryonia.** Short difficult respiration, obliging him to sit erect. Dry cough with stitches in the chest. Violent morning cough, with expectoration of a quantity of mucus. * Sensation when coughing as if the head and chest would fly to pieces. * The patient wants to remain perfectly quiet; the least movement aggravates all his symptoms.

**Carb. veg.** Obstinate hoarseness, particularly in the evening. Tightness in the chest and shortness of breathing. * Severe burning in the chest as if from hot coals. Violent cough with discharge of a quantity of yellowish pus. Cough with vomiting and retching. Stitching pains between the scapula. * Patient craves more air; wants to be fanned all the time.

**Causticum.** Hoarseness and roughness of the throat, particularly in the morning. Short and hacking cough caused by constant tickling in the throat. * When coughing, pain over the hip, involuntary emissions of urine. Loss of voice.

**Cham.** Hoarseness and cough from rattling of mucus in the trachea, the place feeling sore from whence the mucus was detached. * Scraping dry cough from tickling in the larynx, *worse at night,* even during sleep. * One cheek red, and the other pale. * Very impatient, can hardly answer one civilly.

**Hepar s.** Dry, hoarse cough, and roughness in the throat. * Rattling, choking cough, worse after midnight. Hoarse, anxious wheezing breathing, with danger of suffocation when lying down. After exposure to cold west winds.

**Ipecac.** * Rattling of mucus in the bronchial tubes. Suffocative cough with great difficulty of breathing. The chest seems full of phlegm, but does not yield to coughing. * Much nausea and vomiting of mucus.

**Kali bi.** Burning pain in the trachea and bronchi. * Cough, with expectoration of tough, stringy mucus, which can be drawn to the feet.

**Lachesis.** Hoarseness with feeble voice and constriction of the throat. Short, hacking cough, caused by a tingling in the throat. Difficult yellow expectoration. * Larynx and throat painful when touched, and pressure produces violent cough. * Always worse after sleeping and in the afternoon.

**Merc. sol.** Hoarseness and sore throat. Catarrh of the whole mucous membrane. Violent, racking cough, particularly at night, as if it would burst the head and chest. Alternate chilliness and heat. * Cough worse when lying on the right side. * Much perspiration which affords no relief. Thick, yellowish coat on the tongue.

**Nux vom.** Roughness and scraping in the larynx, inducing cough. Dry cough from midnight until morning. Cough with headache as if the skull would burst. Nose stopped up. Fever, but chilliness from slight motion. * Always worse after four o'clock in the morning. * Habitual constipation. After previous use of cough mixtures.

**Phosph.** Complete loss of voice. Painfulness of the larynx. Tightness across the chest. Cough with expectoration of frothy, pale-red or rust-colored mucus. Severe and exhausting cough, which the patient dreads and avoids as long as possible. * Sensation of weakness and emptiness in the abdomen.

**Pulsatilla.** Scraping and dryness in the throat. *Dry cough at night, going off when sitting up in bed.* Loose cough, with copious expectoration of yellow or greenish mucus. * Chilliness even in a warm room. * Hot, dry skin, with little or no thirst. Persons of a mild, tearful disposition.

**Rhus tox.** Roughness in the larynx and soreness in the chest. Cough excited by a tickling under the middle of the sternum, worse from laughing or loud talking. * Rheumatic pains in the bones, worse when at rest. * Worse at night, particularly after midnight.

**Sang. can.** Dryness of the throat and sensation of swelling in the larynx. Severe cough, *with circumscribed redness of the cheeks and pain in the breast.* Fluent coryza and thin diarrhœa. Burning in the hands and feet at night.

**Spongia.** Great dryness in the larynx, with hoarse, hollow, wheezing cough, worse in the evening. Sawing respiration. * The voice frequently gives out when talking or reading aloud.

**Sulphur.** Hoarseness and loss of voice. Sensation as of something creeping in the larynx. Loose cough, with expectoration of thick mucus and soreness in the chest. * Stitches in the chest extending to the back. Pain in the left side. * Frequent weak, faint spells. Constant rattling in the chest. * Lean persons who walk stooping.

**Tartar em.** Large collection of mucus in the bronchial tubes, expectorated with great difficulty. * When the patient coughs, it seems as if much would be expectorated, but nothing comes up. * Nausea and vomiting of much mucus. Great oppression and difficulty of breathing.

**Verat. alb.** Tickling in the lower parts of the

bronchial tubes, inducing cough with slight expectoration. Dry, hollow cough as if proceeding from lower parts of the chest or abdomen. * Rattling of mucus in the chest, but can't get rid of it. * Vomiting with diarrhœa and great prostration.

---

## BURNS AND SCALDS.

**Therapeutics.** Principal remedies.

**1. Cantharides.** In superficial burns or scalds, this is one of the best external applications. Put twenty drops of the *Tincture* in a gill of water and keep the injured parts constantly wet with rags or lint saturated with the solution. After the acute symptoms have subsided, dress the parts with *simple cerate.*

**2. Urtica urens.** This is a remedy of great value in all classes of burns, not only for slight and superficial cases, but in the severe and more deeply penetrating injuries of this kind. It may be applied the same as directed for the use of Cantharides.

**3. Castile Soap.** This has been highly recommended by some in the treatment of burns and scalds. Make a thick salve by mixing it with warm water, spread it upon soft linen or muslin, and apply to the injured part.

**4. Flour and Oil.** This is a good application, and is most always at hand. As soon after the accident as possible, oil the injured surface with sweet or linseed oil, and dust it over with flour from a common dredging-box until it is thickly and completely covered.

**5. Glycerine.** For burns in the mouth, throat, or stomach, this is an excellent remedy. Equal parts of glycerine and water may be taken in spoonful doses, and the mouth and throat gargled with the same. *Urtica urens* taken internally is a remedy of great value in burns of this character.

**Symptomatic indications.**

**Aconite.** Chills, high fever, dry, hot skin and much thirst. * Great fear and anxiety of mind, with much nervous excitability.

**Arsenicum.** Dark, watery, offensive diarrhœa. Rapid and great prostration, with sinking of the vital forces. * Extreme thirst, drinking often, but little at a time. * Great anguish, restlessness, and fear of death.

**Cham.** In *convulsions* arising from severe burns. Becomes almost furious about the pains. * Very impatient, can hardly answer one civilly. Warm sweat about the face and head.

**China.** Extensive suppuration, producing much debility. Painless diarrhœa, of dark watery stools, particularly at night.

**Silicea.** When the ulcer heals but slowly, or proud flesh is disposed to shoot up.

**Sulphur.** There is a strong tendency to the production of proud flesh, and there is no appearance of granulations. Much itching, burning, and inflammation around the ulcers.

---

## CATARRH.

**Therapeutics.** Special indications.

**Aconite.** Mostly in the first stage; chilliness, with burning heat, especially in the head and face. Piercing or throbbing pains in the forehead or temples. Profuse lachrymation. Short, dry cough, from tickling in the larynx. * Fear, anxiety, and great restlessness. * From dry, cold west winds.

**Allium cepa.** * Profuse discharge of water from the eyes, and burning excoriating water from the nose. Terrible laryngeal cough, which compels the patient to grasp the larynx with the hands, for it seems to him that the cough would tear it.

**Ammo. carb.** *Burning of the eyes*, with lachrymation. *Dry coryza*, with stoppage of the nose, especially at night. Dry, *nightly* cough, and stitches in the chest. Frequent chilliness.

**Arsen.** Frequent sneezing, with profuse fluent coryza, and stoppage of the nose. Burning and soreness of the nostrils. Profuse lachrymation and burning in the eyes. Dryness in the mouth and loss of taste. Dry cough with difficult expectoration. Chilliness, particularly after drinking. * Intense thirst, drinking little and often. * Restlessness and prostration.

**Arum. try.** * Coryza, with discharge of burning, ichorous fluid from the nose, excoriating the nostrils and upper lip. Nose stopped up; can only breathe with mouth open. Hoarseness and sore throat. Dry, feverish heat and hot skin.

**Bellad.** Sore throat and hoarseness. * Throbbing headache, worse from motion. Fluent coryza. Ulceration of the nostrils and corners of the mouth. Dry, hoarse cough, especially at night. Alternate chilliness and heat. Swelling and stiffness in the nape of the neck. * Sleepy, but cannot sleep. Aggravation at 3 P. M.

**Bryonia.** Dry coryza, with inflamed and ulcerated nostrils. * Lips parched, dry, and cracked. Dry cough, apparently from the stomach, worse after drinking. * Constipation of hard, dry stools as if burnt. * Patient wants to keep very still. Exceedingly irritable.

**Carb. veg.** Beating or pulsating headache. Burning in the eyes and profuse lachrymation. Stoppage of the nose, particularly in the evening. Fluent coryza, with hoarseness and rawness of the chest. * If the coryza return in the evening.

**Cham.** Fluent, acrid discharge from the nose. Chilliness and feverish heat. * One cheek red and hot, and the other pale and cold. Hoarseness and cough from rattling mucus in the bronchia. * Dry cough, worse at night, even during sleep. * Patient very irritable, can hardly answer one civilly. * Children want to be carried all the time.

**Dulc.** Dry coryza, aggravated in the cold air. Dryness of the mouth without thirst. * The symptoms are aggravated by every cold change, and in wet weather; better when moving about.

**Euphrasia.** * Profuse fluent coryza, with burning acrid tears. Cough only during the day. Ulceration of the margins of the eyelids.

**Gelsem.** Liability to take cold from any change in the weather. Sore throat with pain on swallowing, shooting up into the ear. * Fever without thirst; wants to lie still and rest.

**Hepar s.** Great liability to take cold, especially after the abuse of Mercury. Headache worse by motion. Roughness and scraping sensation in the throat. * Stitches in the throat as if caused by a splinter. * Hoarse croupy cough, the phlegm being loose and choking.

**Ipecac.** Aching pain over the eyes. Fluent coryza, stoppage of the nose and loss of smell. * Rattling of phlegm in the chest, but does not yield to coughing. * Nausea and vomiting of large quantities of mucus. Oppressed breathing as of asthma.

**Kali bic.** Fluent coryza, worse in the evening and in the open air. Flow of acrid water from the nostrils excoriating the parts. * Cough with expectoration of tough phlegm, which can be drawn into long strings. Loss of smell.

**Lachesis.** Fluent coryza, with profuse secretion of mucus and running from the eyes. Dryness of the mouth, with *burning as if from pepper.* Dry cough, shortness of breath and stitches in the chest. * Can bear nothing to touch his throat; it excites the cough and produces a sense of suffocation. * Symptoms worse in the afternoon and after sleeping.

**Merc.** Catarrhal headache. Stitches through the whole head. Burning in the eyes and profuse lachrymation. Pain in the jaws and teeth. * Frequent sneezing and profuse fluent coryza. Feverish heat and redness of the cheeks. Inflamed and *ulcerated tonsils.* Short, dry, fatiguing cough, worse at night. * After sweating at night, the cold is no better. Feels better in a warm room. In epidemic catarrh.

**Nux vom.** Chilliness and feverish heat, pressure and sticking pains in the forehead. * Fluent coryza during the day and dry coryza at night. Dry cough, with headache as if the skull would burst. * Very irritable and wishes to be alone. Constipation, with frequent urging to stool. * Symptoms all worse in the morning.

**Puls.** Discharge of a yellowish, green, thick fetid mucus from the nose. Loss of taste and smell. Toothache and otalgia. Dulness and heaviness in the head, especially in the evening. * Craves fresh cool air, worse in a warm room. * Chilliness even in a warm room. Loose cough, with expectoration of yellow mucus. * Symptoms all worse towards evening. Persons of a mild, tearful disposition.

**Sepia.** Nose swollen and inflamed, with sore and ulcerated nostrils. Obstruction of the nose, and *violent dry* coryza. Loss of smell. Pain in the back and stiffness in the nape of the neck. * Cough, worse in the morning terminating in an effort to vomit. * Great sense of emptiness at the pit of the stomach.

**Sulph.** Catarrh with fluent coryza of clear water. Soreness and pressure in the throat as from a lump. Complete loss of taste and smell. Coldness of the extremities and chilliness. * Frequent weak, faint spells. * Great liability to take cold. * Morning diarrhœa, driving the patient out of bed in great haste.

---

## CHOLERA.

**Therapeutics.** Special indications.

**Aconite.** In the forming stage, where there is great vascular excitement. *Violent heat* and *dryness of the skin.* * Great fear and anxiety of mind, with nervous excitability. Full and frequent pulse. * Vertigo, particularly on raising the head. * Bitter greenish vomiting. Stools whitish, with discharge of lumbrici. * Fear of death, predicts the day he will die.

**Arsen.** * Great anguish, extreme restlessness and fear of death. * Sudden prostration, with sinking of the vital forces. Tongue dry, blackish, and cracked. Violent burning pains in the stomach. Vomiting of watery, slimy, greenish, brownish, or blackish substances; worse after drinking. Frequent watery stools. * Great thirst for cold water, drinks little and often. Skin cold and covered with clammy sweat, or dry and shrivelled.

**Camphor.** In the commencement, when there is great anguish and sudden prostration of strength. Pulse small and rapid. Hands, feet, and skin cold. * Burning pains in the stomach and throat, with cramps in the calves. Painfulness of the pit of the stomach when touched. * Icy coldness and blueness of the face and limbs, even of the tongue. * Half stupid and senseless; he moans and groans in a hoarse husky voice.

**Carb. veg.** Mostly in the *last stage.* * Complete collapse of pulse, the patient lies in a state of asphyxia. The spasms and vomiting have ceased, followed by great debility. Cold breath, cold tongue, or coldness all over. * Livid countenance, hoarse voice, and sunken eyes.

**Croton tig.** Watery discharges from the bowels mixed with whitish flakes. * The discharges always come on after drinking, and are expelled with a sudden gush. Great exhaustion with faintness and vertigo.

**China.** Hippocratic countenance, pointed nose and hollow eyes. Yellowish, blackish or parched tongue. Violent thirst, with a desire to drink often, but little at a time. Spasmodic pains in the stomach. Painless diarrhœa, stools blackish, bilious or whitish. Prostration even unto fainting. * If the disease has supervened upon a great loss of animal fluids.

**Colocynth.** Vomiting, first of food, and afterwards a greenish substance. * Violent constrictive pain in the abdomen as if the intestines were squeezed between stones, *relieved by forcible pressure.* * Terrible cramp-like pains which draw the patient nearly double. Diarrhœa, with thin greenish, slimy, and watery stools. Aggravation after eating or drinking.

**Cuprum me.** Violent vomiting, with colic and diarrhœa. Convulsions of the extremities, especially of the fingers and toes. Rolling of the eyeballs, great restlessness and coldness of the face. Spasmodic colicky pains without vomiting, or vomiting preceded by spasmodic constriction of the chest, arresting the breathing. * Extreme thirst, the liquids descend the throat with a gurgling sound. * Violent cramps in the stomach, fingers, and toes. The vomiting is relieved by drinking cold water.

**Ipecac.** In the early stage, and where *nausea and vomiting* is a prominent symptom. * Vomiting of large quantities of green jelly-like mucus, or black pitch-like substances. Griping pinching in the abdomen, as if grasped with the hands; excited by motion. * Grass-green mucous stools, having the appearance as if fermented. Cramp in the calves, fingers, and toes. Coldness of the face and extremities.

**Phos. acid.** In the commencement, before vomitings set in. Diarrhœa, with whitish, watery, slimy stools, without pain. *Tenacious viscid mucus in the mouth.* * Indifferent, not disposed to talk. Quiet delirium and stupefaction.

**Secale cor.** Face pale and eyes sunken. Dry, thick yellowish-white coating on the tongue. *Unquenchable thirst.* Heat and *burning in the abdomen.* Watery, slimy diarrhœa, or involuntary diarrhœa. The evacuations are preceded by vertigo, anguish, cramps in the calves, rumbling in the abdomen, and nausea. * Great aversion to heat, or to being covered. *Thin, scrawny persons.*

**Verat. alb.** Pale death-like expression of the face. Tongue dry, blackish, and cracked. * Unquenchable thirst for cold drinks. Excessive vomiting of the ingesta with green mucus; also of black bile. * Great weakness after vomiting. Severe cutting pains in the abdomen. Violent diarrhœa with greenish, watery flocculent stools, *followed by rapid prostration.* Cramps in the calves. Small, almost imperceptible, pulse. Hoarse, weak voice, and cold breath. * Cold sweat over the whole body.

---

## CHOLERA INFANTUM.

**Therapeutics.** Special indications.

**Aconite.** In the beginning, when there is dry, hot skin, quick pulse and sleeplessness. Stools green, watery, or white slimy mucus. *Before* and *during* stool, cutting pain and tenesmus. Nausea and vomiting of what has been drunk. * Restlessness, the child turns from side to side.

**Æthusa.** In the worse cases. Stools light-yellow or greenish liquid. *Before* stool, pinching cutting pain in the abdomen. *Violent vomiting of coagulated milk.* * Spasms, with stupor and delirium, clenched thumbs, eyes drawn downward, pupils dilated. Constant thirst; great prostration.

**Ant. crud.** Tongue coated white or yellow. Great dryness of the mouth and lips; no thirst. Violent vomiting of slimy mucus and bile, worse after eating or drinking. Stools watery and profuse. Pain before and during stool. Protrusion of the rectum. * Where the disease was caused by overloading the stomach. * The child cannot bear to be looked at.

**Apis mel.** Tongue dry and shining. No appetite or thirst. Stools *greenish, yellowish,* slimy mucous. *During stool,* griping and tenesmus. Vomiting of bile or thin bitter liquid. Tenderness of the abdomen to pressure. * Aggravation in the morning.

**Arsenicum.** Pale death-like countenance. Skin dry and shrivelled. Stools *thick, dark-green mucous,* or *dark, watery, offensive.* Cutting pain before and tenesmus during stool. * Vomiting immediately after drinking. * Great restlessness, extreme prostration, and the peculiar thirst distinguish this remedy. Aggravation *after midnight.*

**Bellad.** Face pale or flushed. Great dryness of the mouth and lips. Tongue coated white in the middle with red edges. Stools thin green mucous, or bloody mucous. Tenesmus during and after stool. *Delirium, worse during and just after sleep, with desire to get out of bed.* * Sleepy, but cannot sleep. * Child cries out suddenly, and ceases just as suddenly. * Sudden starting and jumping during sleep.

**Benzoic ac.** *Fetid, watery, white stools, very copious* and exhausting. *During* stool, much pressing or straining. * Strong-smelling urine, mostly dark-colored. Troublesome and dry hacking cough. Tongue coated with white mucus, or ulcerated.

**Borax.** Pale clay-colored appearance of the face. Aphthæ in the mouth and on the tongue. *Light yellow,* *slimy mucous*, or greenish, watery stools. Pinching pain in the abdomen. * Fear of falling from downward motion, even during sleep. * Easily startled at sudden noise, with anxious screams.

**Bryonia.** Dry parched lips and mouth. Thirst for *large quantities* of water at long intervals. * Vomiting of food soon after taking it, undigested. Stools brown, thin fecal, or undigested. Previous to stool, the child cries out with pain, and cannot bear to be moved, as it increases the suffering. * Gets faint and sick on sitting up. Symptoms worse in the morning. If caused from *cold drinks*, or from getting *overheated.*

**Calc. carb.** Children with *large heads and open fontanelles — scrofulous.* Swollen, distended abdomen, with emaciation and good appetite. Skin dry and shrivelled. Stools whitish and watery, or *chalk-like ; undigested.* Vomiting of sour substances, particularly of milk. * Profuse sweat on the head when sleeping, * Cold damp feet.

**Carb. veg.** Great paleness, or gray-yellow color of the face. Dryness of the mouth without thirst. Stools *light-colored; involuntary; putrid; cadaverous smelling.* Mostly in the last stage, and where the vital powers are greatly exhausted. Restlessness and anxiety, worse towards evening. * Emission of large quantities of flatus, inodorous, or putrid.

**Cham.** Redness and heat of the face, sometimes *one cheek red and the other pale.* Tongue coated thick yellow, or white. Sour vomiting of food, or slimy substances. *Green, watery, corroding* stools with colic; also mixed *white and yellow mucous*, like chopped eggs. Colic *before* and *during* stool. * The child is very fretful, and wants to be carried all the time.

**China.** Tympanitic distention of the abdomen. Stools *yellow, watery*, undigested, painless, or blackish and offensive. Before stool, colic which is relieved by bending double. Patient worse *after eating*, and at night. * Great weakness and inclination to sweat. Emission of much flatulence. * Worse every other day.

**Cina.** Children that are troubled with worms. Paleness of the face, particularly around the nose and mouth. * Disposition to pick and bore at the nose. White papescent stools. * White, turbid, or jelly-like urine. *Restless sleep, frequent changing position*, and *waking with cries.* Grinding of the teeth during sleep.

**Croton tig.** *Dry parched lips.* Nausea and vomiting of water, mucus, and bile, especially after drinking. Yellow watery, dark green, or greenish-yellow stools, *coming out like a shot.* * Worse after drinking, while nursing. *Great prostration after stool.*

**Dulc.** Dry heat of the skin, and violent thirst for cold drink. Stools yellowish, green, watery, or whitish. Colic before and during stool. * The child gets worse at every cold change in the weather, or from exposure to cold air. After taking cold or getting wet.

**Gumm. gut.** Loud rumbling and gurgling in the bowels. Stools *thin yellow fecal*, or *dark green* and *offensive.* * Sudden expulsion of the stool, coming out in a gush. Nausea and vomiting after eating or drinking. The child seems to crave food, but little satisfies it. Aphthæ in the mouth.

**Ipecac.** Pale face, with blue margins around the eyes. Yellowish or white coated tongue. * Almost constant *nausea and vomiting.* The child throws up its food, and large quantities of green mucus. Stools *grass-green mucous*, or white, fermented. Colic and sick stomach *before* and *during* stool. * After vomiting inclination to sleep.

**Laurocerasus.** Sunken countenance ; livid, grayish-yellow complexion. Eyes staring or lightly closed. Tongue white and dry, with violent thirst. Pulse slow, *irregular*, or *imperceptible.* Stools green, liquid, mucous, involuntary. Cutting pain in the abdomen before and tenesmus after stool. * *Rattling sound of liquids when passing through the œsophagus.*

**Magnesia c.** Face dirty dark yellow. No appetite, violent thirst, inclination to vomit. * Stools green and slimy, like the scum of a frog-pond, smelling sour. Before stool, *cutting and pinching* in the abdomen. Worse in hot weather, and during dentition.

**Merc.** *Dry lips*, with ulcerated corners of the mouth. Tongue *coated as with fur.* Vomiting and empty retching. Violent thirst. Stools yellow, the color of sulphur, sometimes green, slimy, or bloody. * Colic before, and *violent tenesmus during and after* stool. * Great tenderness over the pit of the stomach and abdomen. Cold clammy sweats, especially at night.

**Nux mos.** *Great languor;* cold, dry skin, little or no thirst. Colic, worse after eating or drinking; *relieved by the application of moist heat.* Stools *thin yellow* (like beaten or stirred eggs), undigested, watery, slimy. Colic *before*, and urging during stool. * *Great drowsiness and dulness of sense.* Worse at night, and in cool damp weather.

**Nux vom.** Tongue coated thick yellowish-white. Swelling of the gums, and fetid ulcers in the mouth. Vomiting of sour-smelling mucus. Frequent, small, watery, slimy, *dark-colored, mucous stools.* Colic before and *violent straining at stool;* relief after stool. * After gastric medicines and prolonged drugging. Worse in the early morning.

**Phosphorus.** Pale, sickly complexion; hollow eyes, with blue margins around the same; dry tongue, coated with white mucus; *thirst* for cold drinks. *Vomiting* of what has been drunk as soon as it *becomes warm in the stomach.* Stools *white watery,* containing little lumps *like grains of tallow;* undigested. * Watery stools, pouring away as from a hydrant. Worse in the morning, and from lying on the left side.

**Phos. ac.** Blue margins around the eyes; violent thirst; loss of appetite; profuse perspiration at night. Stools *whitish, watery,* light yellow, *painless.* * The disease is not marked by *much debility,* though it may continue a long time.

**Podophyl.** Moaning during sleep, with half-closed eyes, and rolling the head from side to side. *Gagging or empty retching.* Stools watery, with meal-like sediment; dark-yellow mucous, *smelling like carrion.* * Profuse watery, painless stools, very exhaustive. * Prolapsus ani during stool. Worse in the morning, and after eating and drinking.

**Puls.** Tongue coated with tenacious mucus. *Thirstlessness.* * Stools very changeable, no two alike, worse at night. Before stool, *rumbling* in the bowels, during stool *chilliness.*

**Secal. cor.** Face pale, eyes sunken and surrounded by blue margins. Dry, thick yellowish-white coating on the tongue. Easy, painless vomiting, without effort, very exhausting. Stools *watery and slimy, involuntary.* Before stool, cutting and rumbling in the abdomen; great exhaustion during and after stool. * Great aversion to heat, or to being covered. * Thin, scrawny children, with shrivelled skin.

**Silicea.** * Children with large heads and open fontanelles — scrofulous. *Profuse perspiration on the head,* particularly during sleep. Stools liquid, slimy, frothy, or bloody mucous. Colic, and distention of the abdomen. Where the disease is complicated with a *psoric derangement.*

**Sulphur.** The child is very drowsy through the day and wakeful at night. Stools very changeable, attended with pain, or no pain at all; *worse in the early morning.* * Stools very excoriating. When there are repeated relapses, or the case seems to linger a long while.

**Thuja oc.** Great desire for cold drinks; rapid exhaustion; oppressed breathing; great emaciation. * Stools *pale-yellow watery,* very copious, and gushing out like water from a bung-hole. Aggravation in the morning, and after vaccination.

**Verat. alb.** Cold sweat on the forehead. Lips dry and dark-colored. * Vomiting, excited by the smallest quantities of liquids, with great prostration. The least motion increases the vomiting. Stools *greenish watery, with flakes.* Before stool, severe colic; during stool, *cold sweat on the forehead.* * Violent thirst for large quantities of cold water. Pulse almost imperceptible.

---

## COLIC.

**Therapeutics.** Special indications.

**Aconite.** Inflammatory colic involving the bladder. Difficult and scanty emissions of urine. Great sensitiveness of the abdomen. Intolerable cutting pains in the belly, so violent that he screams, tosses about, and is almost beside himself. * Great fear and anxiety of mind, with nervous excitability.

**Aloes**. Violent cutting pains in the bowels; or beating, boring, and stinging in the region of the umbilicus. Dull, heavy headache, with dull pains in the liver. * Loud gurgling in the abdomen, as of water running out of a bottle. *Large and prominent hemorrhoids.*

**Ars. alb**. Severe cutting, or spasmodic, drawing pains; or a sensation as if the *intestines had become twisted.* Violent burning pains in the stomach. * Extreme thirst, drinks little and often. * Great restlessness, anxiety, and fear of death. *Prostration* and cold sweat.

**Bell.** Pad-shaped protrusion of the transverse colon. * Clutching pain in the abdomen as if seized with claws. *Constriction of the abdomen around the umbilicus, as if a ball or lump would form.* External pressure and bending double relieves somewhat. * Periodical pains, which come on suddenly, and cease as suddenly. Mostly worse in the afternoon, and after sleeping.

**Bryo.** Hard swelling around the umbilicus, and under the hypochondrium. Spasms of the stomach. Painful twisting around the umbilicus, with frequent stitches. * Wants to keep perfectly still, as the least motion or pressure increases the pain. Vomiting of bitter bile and water, particularly after drinking. Nausea and fainting on sitting up. * Hard, dry stools, as if burnt.

**Carb. veg.** Great fulness in the abdomen as if it would burst. Crampy pain in the left side of the epigastrium, more towards the back. Incarcerated flatus in different parts of the abdomen. Frequent eructations affording no relief. * Constant pressure downwards in the abdomen. Audible rumbling in the bowels, and belching of sour, rancid food. * Prostration, hippocratic face, with coldness of the extremities. *Worse from 4 to 6* P. M.

**Cham.** *Flatulent colic*, the abdomen being distended like a drum. Continual drawing, tearing pains in the abdomen, with a sensation as if the bowels were rolled up in a ball. Pressing toward the abdominal ring, as if a hernia would protrude. *Vomiting of sour food*, or of *slimy substances*. * Very impatient, can hardly answer one civilly. * Children want to be carried all the time. * He becomes almost furious about the pains.

**China.** Flatulent colic, with thirst. Tympanitic distention of the abdomen. Violent cutting, pinching pains about the navel, relieved by bending double. * The abdomen feels full and tight as if stuffed. If the disease was caused by eating fruit or drinking new beer. After exhausting illness, or loss of vital fluids.

**Cocc.** *Violent spasms of the stomach*, with a *griping-lacerating!*sensation. Contraction of the abdomen, with a downward and outward pressure. Flatulent colic at midnight; belching relieves. * Abdomen distended, and feels as if full of sharp stones when moving.

**Coffea.** Insupportable *labor-like* pains in the abdomen. Sensation as if the bowels would be cut to pieces; horrible cries and grinding of the teeth. * The patient becomes desperate on account of the pains. Cannot bear to be touched, the parts are so sensitive. * Great excitability.

**Colo.** *Violent cutting, constrictive or spasmodic pains.* * Feeling in the whole abdomen as if the *intestines were being squeezed between stones, compelling one to bend double*, worse in any other position. Great restlessness, moaning, and lamentation. After violent indignation, or after the abuse of opium.

**Cup. met.** Violent spasms in the abdomen and in the upper and lower limbs, by spells. Cutting and lacerating in the bowels. * A violent piercing pain, as if a knife were penetrating through from the umbilicus to the back. *Fearful cries as if he were being killed.* Convulsive movements and distortions of the limbs.

**Ignatia.** *Periodical spasms* in the abdomen in sensitive and hysterical persons. Colic, first pinching, afterwards sticking in one side of the abdomen. Nightly flatulent colic, and much rumbling in the bowels. * Sadness and sighing, with a weak, empty feeling at the pit of the stomach.

**Ipecac.** Horrid, indescribable pain and sick feeling in the stomach. Cutting and pinching (as if grasping with the hands) around the umbilicus, worse by motion, and better by rest. * Constant nausea, stooping causes him to vomit. *After vomiting, inclination to sleep.*

**Merc.** Very sensitive over the pit of the stomach and abdomen. Pinching pains in the abdomen, during which he is *attacked with chilliness and shuddering.* Frequent urging to stool; slimy diarrhœa. * Cold clammy sweat on the thighs and legs.

**Nux vom.** Cramp-like pains in the stomach, with pressure towards the thorax. *Pressure in the stomach as from a stone.* Cutting, pinching pains, with desire to vomit and belch. Flatulent colic, with distention of the bowels. * Frequent urging to stool, without effect. Persons of a *malicious, irritable disposition; high livers, and the victims of drug medication.*

**Plumb. met.** *Violent colic,* with *sunken abdomen.* * Terrible contractive pains, drawing in the abdomen to the back. Constriction of the intestines, the navel and anus are violently drawn in. * Obstinate constipation, fæces lumpy, and packed together like sheep's dung. Suppression of urine from paralysis of the bladder.

**Puls.** Putrid, bitter taste, especially after taking food or drink. Aching drawing pains in the pit of the stomach. Eructations tasting of the ingesta. Painful sensitiveness of the abdominal walls. Frequent loose stools very changeable, worse at night. Patient can't bear to be covered, and craves fresh cold air. If caused from eating *rich greasy food.* * Persons of a mild, tearful disposition.

**Sulph.** Painful sensitiveness in the abdomen, as if all the parts were raw and sore. Pain as if something would be torn out. Hemorrhoidal colic. Thin, lean persons, who walk stooping. After eating sweet things.

**Verat. alb.** Pain here and there in the abdomen, as if cut with knives. Terrible colic (cutting pains), with *violent nausea and vomiting.* Great thirst for large quantities of cold drinks. Anxiety, fear, and despair. * Cold sweat over the whole body. *Great weakness, with very feeble pulse.*

---

## CONSTIPATION.

**Therapeutics.** Special indications.

**Alumina.** Great inactivity of the rectum, as if paralyzed. Hard and difficult stool attended with pain in the rectum. * Stools very hard, knotty, and scant. Sensation of pricking and excoriation in the rectum after an evacuation. * Much pressing and straining to pass even a soft stool, so inactive is the rectum.

**Agaricus.** Stools *first hard and knotty*, afterwards loose, and finally diarrhœic. Itching and tingling of the anus, as of ascarides. Gastric derangements, *with sharp stitches in the region of the liver.* * Itching, burning, and redness of the feet and hands, as if frozen.

**Ammo. mur.** Whining, peevish, insociable mood. Empty eructations, and painful stitches in the left hypochondrium, early in the morning. Disposition to constipation; *stools large and hard*, followed by soft stools. * Large hard stools, crumbling as they pass from the anus.

**Anacar.** Frequent and ineffectual urging to stool. * The rectum feels as if stopped up with a plug. If the expulsion does not take place soon, a painful twisting is felt across the abdomen. Stools, first loose, afterwards hard and of a very pale color.

**Ant. crud.** Hard stool with very difficult expulsion and much previous straining. Alternate diarrhœa and constipation of aged persons. * A sensation as if a copious stool would take place, when only flatus is expelled; finally a very hard stool is voided. Protrusion of the rectum during stool.

**Apis mel.** Pain in the eyeballs and forehead.

Inability to fix the thoughts on any subject. Tenderness of the abdomen to pressure. No stool for several days, then very difficult, with stinging pains in the abdomen. * Sensation in the abdomen as if something would break if much effort was made to void the stool.

**Bell.** Constipation, with tendency of blood to the head. When stooping, the blood rushes to the head followed by giddiness. * Violent throbbing and stitching pains, particularly in the forehead. Plethoric individuals, or persons with blonde hair and red complexion.

**Bryo.** Lips dry and parched, with much thirst for large quantities of water. Frequent eructations, especially after a meal; food is vomited immediately after eating. Headache as if the skull would split, aggravated by the least motion. * Hard, dry stools as if burnt. *Irritable mood.*

**Calc. carb.** * Stools large, hard, and sometimes only partially digested. After stool, a gloomy feeling in the head. * Cold damp feet. Women who suffer with *profuse and too frequent menses.* Scrofulous diathesis.

**Caust.** Frequent and unsuccessful desire to pass stool, accompanied with pain, anxiety, and redness of the face. * Stools tough, light-colored, whitish, *shining like grease.* Soreness in the anus and rectum when walking.

**Chelido.** Suitable to persons subject to hepatic diseases. Sallow, jaundiced complexion. * Constant pain under the lower inner angle of the right shoulder-blade. * Stools like sheep's dung.

**Graph.** Constipation with much tenesmus and stitches in the rectum. * Stools hard and knotty, the lumps being united by mucous threads. Sometimes a large quantity of mucus is expelled with the stool. Unhealthy skin. * Itching blotches over the body, which emit a glutinous fluid.

**Ignatia.** Difficult stool, causing prolapsus of the rectum. Anxious desire for stool, with inactivity of the rectum. Constipation from taking cold, or from riding in a carriage. * After stool, a violent stabbing stitch, from the anus upwards into the rectum. * Full of grief, with a weak, empty feeling in the stomach. Hemorrhoids, the tumors prolapse with every stool.

**Iodine.** In the constipation of scrofulous people, with a low cachectic state of the system. * Stools hard, knotty, and dark-colored. Chronic headache, and vertigo, especially in old people. Throbbing in the head at every motion.

**Kali carb.** Constipation every other day, with painful drawing in the abdomen. *Inactivity of the rectum.* The stools are too large, and there is a sensation as if the rectum were too weak to expel it. * Distress with stitching colicky pains an hour or two before stool. Aged persons inclined to be fleshy.

**Lycop.** Ineffectual urging, particularly in the evening. Stools *very hard, scant, and passed with great difficulty.* Sensation after stool as if much remained behind. Acidity and heartburn, with *great drowsiness* after dinner. Much fermentation as if a yeast-pot were in the abdomen. * Loud rumbling and gurgling in the bowels. * Red sediment like sand in the urine.

**Mag. mur.** Frequent and severe pressure on the rectum with colic. Stool hard and knotty, with pain in the rectum when passing it. * Large difficult stools crumbling when passing from the anus. Throbbing in the pit of the stomach, with dulness of the head.

**Nitric ac.** Painless constipation. Stools *hard, dry, and scant.* Difficult, irregular stool, with much pressing. Headache; it feels as if surrounded by a tight bandage. *Sour or bitter taste after eating;* sour eructations. Excessive flatulence. * Fetid and strong smelling urine, like that of horses. Antidotes all diseases having a *mercurial origin.*

**Nux vom.** Stools *large, hard,* and passed with great difficulty. * Sensation as if the anus were closed, or too narrow. Frequent eructations of sour or bitter fluids. Feeling of fulness in the stomach soon after eating. * Sensation as if a stone, or lump of lead were in the stomach. Constipation from *sedentary habits,* and of pregnant women. Where the disease has been induced by the use of rich or highly-seasoned food, drastic medicines, or prolonged drugging. *Frequent urging to stool.*

**Opium.** Torpor of the bowels, after chronic diarrhœa, or from abuse of cathartics. Costiveness for weeks, with loss of appetite. * Stools of nothing but *small hard black balls.* * Constipation from fright or fear. *Paralysis* of the intestines.

**Phos.** For persons with phthisical constitutions, lean and slender. * Stools long, narrow, and hard, like a dog's: very difficult to expel. Alternate diarrhœa and constipation of old people. * Belching up large quantities of wind after eating. Very sleepy after meals, especially after dinner.

**Plumb. met.** Constipation with violent colic. * Stools composed of little hard black-brown balls, resembling sheep's dung. A sense of constriction in the sphincter ani, with ineffectual urging.

**Puls.** Constipation produced by derangement of the stomach, consequent upon eating too much *rich, greasy food.* Obstinate constipation; also, alternate diarrhœa and constipation. Adapted to females, or persons of a mild, gentle, tearful disposition.

**Ruta.** Hard, scanty stool, almost like sheep's-dung. * Frequent urging to stool, with protrusion of the rectum. Great difficulty in voiding the stool on account of the protrusion of the rectum. Constipation following mechanical injuries.

**Sarsap.** Obstinate constipation, with urging to urinate. Desire for stool, with contraction of the intestines and pressure from above downwards. * Feeling as if the bowels would be pressed out during stool. Frequent but scanty emissions of urine, especially at night.

**Sepia.** Stools hard and knotty, sometimes mingled with mucus, with cutting pains in the rectum. * Sense of weight or of a lump in the anus, not relieved by stool. * Especially suited to pregnant women, or to females suffering from uterine difficulties.

**Silicea.** Constipation of difficult stools, as if the *rectum had not power to expel them.* * After much effort and straining, the stool *recedes back into the rectum* after having been partially expelled. Constipation of females, particularly before and during menstruation; also of infants and scrofulous children.

**Sulph.** Chronic constipation. Stools hard and lumpy, mixed with mucus, followed by burning pain in the anus and rectum. Hard, knotty stools, insufficient, accompanied by hemorrhoids. The *first effort at stool is often very painful,* compelling the patient to desist. Flashes of heat, and throbbing headache. * Constant heat on top of the head. * Frequent weak, faint spells.

**Sulph. ac.** *Hard, knotty stools, streaked with blood, very fetid.* Pain during stool as if the rectum would be torn. Pinching in the sides of the abdomen, and prickings in the anus during stool. * Much debility, with a tremulous sensation over the whole body, without trembling.

**Thuya.** *Violent pain in the rectum during stool.* Discharge of large, hard, brown fæces, in balls, streaked with blood. Painful contraction in the anus and rectum, followed by tearing pains in the bowels. * Copious and frequent urination, with burning in the urethra.

**Verat. alb.** Chronic constipation, particularly of infants. Stools of large size and very hard. Inactivity of the rectum, it seems as if paralyzed. * Much straining, with cold perspiration on the forehead. * Great exhaustion and faintness after stool.

**Zinc. met.** Constipation, with *hard, dry, insufficient stool, with much straining,* and rumbling in the bowels. * Trembling of the hands, with coldness of the extremities. * Chronic sick headache, and great weakness of sight. *Fidgety feeling in the feet and legs;* he must move them constantly.

---

## COUGH.

**Therapeutics.** Special indications.

**Aconite.** *Short, dry cough,* arising from a constant tickling in the larynx, excited by smoking, or drinking, and *at night.* Stitches in the chest, hindering respiration. Cannot breathe freely, the lungs feel as if they would not expand. * Persons of a plethoric habit, and where the disease was induced by a cold west wind.

**Arnica.** *Dry, short, and tickling* cough, particularly in the *morning after rising*. Also for a cough with expectoration of mucus and coagulated blood. *Stitching pain* in the *side of the chest*, increased by coughing. * The chest and abdomen feel as if bruised, with shortness of breath.

**Arsen.** Dry cough, as if caused by the smoke of sulphur, with a sense of suffocation; aggravated by drinking, at night after midnight, and in the cold air. Cough with scanty and difficult expectoration, sometimes with blood-streaked mucus. Anxious and oppressive shortness of breath, particularly when going up stairs. * Anxiety, restlessness; thirst for cold water, but drinks little.

**Arum tri.** *Loose cough*, particularly in children and aged persons, where there is inability to expectorate the accumulated mucus. Hoarseness; throat sore and feels as if excoriated. * Discharge of a gleety fluid from the nose, excoriating the nostrils and upper lip.

**Bell.** Dry spasmodic cough, worse at night and from motion. Night-cough, frequently waking the patient from sleep, with catarrh and stitches in the chest. Sensation as if *down or dust were in the throat, causing a constant tickling in the larynx*, with irresistible desire to cough. * Redness and heat of the face, with throbbing headache.

**Bryo.** Dry cough, preceded by a tickling or creeping in the pit of the stomach, and vomiting of the ingesta during the cough. Violent cough, particularly in the morning, with expectoration of a quantity of mucus. Stitches in the chest, when coughing or breathing deep. Sensation when coughing, as if the head and chest would fly to pieces. * Dry hard stools as if burnt. Is very irritable and disposed to be angry.

**Calc. c.** *Dry* cough, especially in the evening and after midnight, with palpitation of the heart. Also cough *early in the morning, with yellow expectoration.* Tightness in the chest, as if there was not room to breathe. General weakness; great fatigue when walking. * When going up stairs he is out of breath and has to sit down. * Cold damp feet.

**Caps.** *Dry cough*, worse in the evening and during the night. Headache and inclination to vomit during the cough. Throbbing pain in the chest. * Shuddering and chilliness in the back.

**Carb. veg.** *Short dry cough*, caused by a tickling in the throat, which frequently excites vomiting and retching. Also for a violent cough, with expectoration of a quantity of yellowish pus, accompanied by stitches in the left side of the chest.

**Caust.** *Short dry cough*, caused by a constant tickling in the throat without expectoration. * Cough with involuntary emissions of urine. Soreness of the chest when coughing. Hoarseness, particularly in the morning, with dry cough.

**Cham.** *Dry tickling cough*, worse at night, even during sleep, especially in children after taking cold. * One cheek red and the other pale. * Patient very irritable, can hardly answer one civilly. * Children are very cross and want to be carried all the time.

**China.** Dry hacking cough, as if caused by the vapor of sulphur, without any expectoration. Cough excited by laughing, talking, drinking, or by deep inspiration. Also cough *with expectoration of clear tenacious mucus*, or blood-streaked mucus. * After hemorrhage from the lungs, and other debilitating losses.

**Cina.** *Dry spasmodic cough*, particularly in children *troubled with worms*. The child starts suddenly as if it would loose its senses, gasps for breath, coughs and gags as if something was in his throat. * Continually picking and boring at the nose. * The urine turns milky after standing but a short time.

**Dros.** *Loose cough*, with expectoration of yellowish mucus, and hoarse voice, having a deep base sound. Pain in the chest and under the ribs when coughing, obliging the patient to hold the painful part with the hands. Vomiting of food, after which, of phlegm and water. Worse at night when lying in bed, after singing, laughing, &c.

**Hepar s.** *Croupy cough*, with loose rattling of

phlegm in the windpipe. * Rattling, choking cough, worse after midnight. Also, for a *dry hoarse cough*, worse in the morning. * Cannot bear to be uncovered, the least exposure to cold excites the cough. Anxious, hoarse, wheezing respiration.

**Hyos.** * *Dry spasmodic cough*, especially at night and when lying down, relieved by sitting up. Bluish color of the face, twitching and jactitation of the muscles over the whole body. Hysterical females and young girls.

**Ignatia.** *Dry spasmodic cough*, as if caused by the vapor of sulphur or dust in the throat. Constant hacking cough in the evening in bed. * Full of grief, with weak, empty feeling at the pit of the stomach. * Stitches in hemorrhoidal tumors during every cough.

**Ipecac.** *Dry cough*, produced by a tickling in the upper part of the larynx. Suffocative cough, *with rattling of mucus in the bronchial tubes when breathing.* Children when coughing almost suffocate, and become purple in the face. * Much nausea, and vomiting of tenacious, white, glary mucus. Green, watery, or fermented stools, with nausea and colic.

**Kali bi.** *Loose cough*, with rattling in the chest. Cough with thick, heavy expectoration of bluish, lumpy mucus. * Cough, with expectoration of *tough viscid mucus*, which can be *drawn out in long strings.* During the cough, pain in the sternum, darting through between the shoulders.

**Lachesis.** *Short, dry cough*, caused by a tickling in the throat. * The slightest pressure on the larynx causes a violent cough and a sense of suffocation. Larynx and throat painful to touch ; *cannot bear anything on the neck.* Soreness in the chest and stitches in the side, worse when coughing. Worse during the day, and *after sleeping*.

**Lyco.** Cough with gray, salt expectoration, and great weakness of the stomach. Morning cough with *green expectoration* and violent pain in the side. Also cough with thick white-yellowish expectoration. Stitches in the left side of the chest during an inspiration, * Fan-like motion of the alæ nasi. Constipation of large, hard, difficult stools. * Red sediment like sand in the urine.

**Merc.** *Dry cough*, which sounds as if the whole inside of the chest were dry. Cough with expectoration of yellowish mucus; sometimes attended with spitting of blood. * Much perspiration affording no relief. Patient worse at night and in damp, rainy weather.

**Nux vom.** *Dry cough*, caused by a rough, scraping, acrid sensation in the throat. Dry cough in the evening and at night, with slight expectoration through the day. Cough with pain in the head, as if the skull would burst, or a sensation as if bruised in the region of the stomach. * Constipation of large, hard, difficult stools. Aggravation in the morning, and from physical or mental exertion.

**Phos.** Mostly a *dry cough*, arising from a tickling in the throat and chest, and where it is excited by reading aloud, talking, laughing, or drinking. * Dry tickling cough in the evening, with *tightness across the chest.* * Long, narrow, hard stools, very difficult to expel. Tall, slender persons, with phthisical constitutions.

**Phos. ac.** Cough with expectoration of yellow phlegm, only in the morning. Cough with purulent, very offensive expectoration. Headache when coughing, with nausea and vomiting of food, or with involuntary emissions of urine.

**Puls.** *Dry cough* during the night, *going off when sitting up in bed.* Also, a loose cough, with yellowish, greenish, or bitter expectoration, which is discharged easily. * Morning cough with much yellow, salty, bitter, disgusting expectoration; sometimes attended with vomiting. Stitching pains in the sides of the chest, particularly when lying down. * All the symptoms worse towards evening. Persons of a mild tearful disposition.

**Silicea.** For a *dry* or *loose* cough, with expectoration of a quantity of transparent mucus. Dry hacking cough, with soreness of the chest. Also cough, with *vomiting of much purulent matter.* Aching in the sternum, towards the stomach. Want of vital heat; inclines to be cold. * Constipation, the stools *recede after having been partially expelled.*

**Stann.** *Loose cough,* with rattling breathing. * Cough, with profuse greenish expectoration of a disagreeable sweetish taste. Also cough with yellowish expectoration having a putrid taste. After every cough, a sore feeling in the chest and trachea. Scrofulous or phthisical subjects.

**Sulph.** *Dry cough,* with hoarseness and dryness in the throat. Also, for a *loose cough,* with expectoration of greenish lumps having a sweetish taste. * Much rattling of mucus in the lungs, cough worse in the morning. Dry, scaly, unhealthy skin. * Lean persons, who walk stooping.

**Tartar em.** *Loose cough, without* expectoration. Rattling or hollow cough, worse at night, with suffocative spells. * Throat full of phlegm, sweat breaks out at every coughing spell. * Nausea and vomiting of large quantities of mucus. *Thirst day and night.*

**Verat. alb.** *Deep hollow* cough, caused by a *tickling low down in the bronchial tubes,* with slight expectoration. Cough with yellow expectoration, and a bruised pain in the chest after coughing. Violent cough with blueness of the face, and involuntary emissions of urine. *Excessive weakness.*

---

## CROUP.

**Therapeutics.** Special indications.

**Aconite.** *First stage,* when there is high fever, dry hot skin and *great restlessness.* On attempting to swallow, the child cries as if from soreness and pain in the throat. * Loud breathing during expiration, but not during inspiration. * Every expiration ends with a hoarse, hacking cough.

**Ammo. caus.** Deep, weak voice; can scarcely utter a word. Cough with copious expectoration of mucus, especially after drinking. *Difficult, labored, rattling breathing;* stertorous breathing. Spasms of chest and suffocative fits.

**Bell.** Heat of the head; *face flushed and eyes red.* Great soreness of the larynx, and when touched the child seems as if it would suffocate. Bright redness of the fauces. Dry, barking, spasmodic cough. Short, anxious inspirations with moaning. * Sleepiness, but cannot sleep. * Starting and jumping during sleep.

**Bromine.** Great oppression and difficulty of breathing; *child gasping for air. Spasm of the larynx causing suffocation.* Dry, hoarse, spasmodic cough, with wheezing, rattling respiration, impeding speech. * Formation of a false membrane in the larynx and trachea. Pulse frequent, feeble, and tremulous. Worse from evening until midnight.

**Cham.** Catarrhal croup, where there is *much hoarseness, wheezing and rattling of mucus in the trachea.* Dry, short, croupy cough, worse at night, even during sleep. * The child is very cross, and wants to be carried all the time. * One cheek red and the other pale.

**Hepar s.** Croup, with *loose, rattling, choking cough;* the air-passages seem clogged with mucus. Violent fits of coughing as if the child would suffocate or vomit; slight nervous or vascular excitement. * The child cannot bear to be uncovered, and coughs whenever any part of the body gets cold. Great drowsiness and profuse sweat.

**Iodine.** * Soreness and pain in the throat and chest, which the child manifests by grasping the parts with the hand. *Dry, short, hacking cough,* with great difficulty of breathing. *Membranous croup, with wheezing, sawing respiration.* * Face pale and cold; voice deep, rough, and hoarse.

**Kali bi.** In *true membranous croup.* The disease approaches gradually; at first, there is slight dyspnœa, with hoarse, croupy cough; as it progresses, the difficulty of breathing increases, and the air as it passes through the trachea, *sounds as though it were passing through a metallic tube.* Hoarse, dry, barking cough. Tonsils and larynx red, swollen, and covered with a pseudo-membrane. Head inclined backwards; violent wheezing and rattling in the trachea, heard at a distance.

**Lachesis.** In far advanced cases, where there is

threatened paralysis of the lungs. Patches of exudation on the fauces. * Larynx very painful to touch, the slightest pressure causes spasmodic suffocative cough. Can bear nothing tight about the neck. Tossing about and moaning during sleep. * *Distressing aggravation after sleeping.*

**Phos.** Great hoarseness with painfulness of the larynx, impeding speech. * Cannot talk on account of pain in the larynx. * Trembling of the whole body while coughing. Shortness of breath, which otherwise has a natural sound. Hoarseness after croup, and where there is a tendency to relapse.

**Spong.** * *Non-membranous* croup, where there is a rough, crowing, and barking cough. *Slow, loud, wheezing* and *sawing respiration*, or suffocative fits, with inability to breathe except with the head bent backwards. * The stridulous respiratory sound is heard during *inspiration*, and the cough which is *dry*, is excited only during the respiratory act. Fluent coryza, and sometimes sneezing, with *saliva drivelling* from the mouth.

**Tartar em.** In the advanced stages of croup, where there are indications of paralysis of the pneumogastric nerves. * With every cough, a sound as if a large quantity of mucus were lodged in the bronchial tubes, while none is expectorated. Respiration very difficult, short, hoarse, shrill, or whistling. The chest expands with great difficulty; head thrown back, much *anxiety and prostration.* Forehead, and sometimes the whole body, covered with cold perspiration.

---

## CYSTITIS, ETC.

The symptoms characterizing inflammation of the bladder are so closely related to those of Dysuria, Irritable bladder, Retention of urine, &c., that we will include under one head the appropriate remedies for these several morbid conditions.

**Therapeutics.** Principal remedies.

**Acon.** Dry, hot skin, intense thirst and great

restlessness. Frequent and violent urging to urinate, with difficult and scanty emissions of deep red turbid urine. * Retention of urine, with stitches in the kidneys. Painfulness of the region of the bladder. * Great fear and anxiety of mind, with nervous excitability.

**Arnica.** When the disturbance arises from mechanical injury. Retention of urine, with tenesmus of the neck of the bladder. Urging, the urine dropping out involuntary. *Brown urine, with brick-red sediment.* * Pain in the small of the back as if bruised.

**Apis m.** Burning, smarting pain before and after urination. Stinging pains in the urethra during micturition; the *urine dark-colored and scanty.* * Incontinence of urine, with great irritation of the parts; worse at night and when coughing. * Sensation as if something in the abdomen would break, if too much effort was made to void the urine.

**Bell.** Difficult micturition, the urine being passed drop by drop, with frequent urging. The urine is yellow and turbid, or the color of gold; sometimes depositing a reddish sediment. * Constant dribbling of urine, wholly involuntary; also enuresis with profuse perspiration. Sharp stitches low down in the abdomen, in the direction of the perineum. * Pains come on suddenly, and cease just as suddenly. Feeling in the back as if it would break.

**Camph.** Burning heat in the region of the bladder. Retention of urine with constant pressure on the bladder and desire to urinate. *Red thick urine,* depositing a thick sediment. Burning in the urethra during micturition. * Strangury, especially if caused by the abuse of cantharides. Coldness of the extremities, with cramp in the calves.

**Cann. in.** Inflammation of the bladder. Painful discharge by drops of *bloody urine.* Darting stitches in the posterior portion of the urethra. * Violent burning in the urethra during and after micturition. Drawing pain from the region of the kidneys to the inguinal glands, with anxious and sick feeling in the pit of the stomach.

**Canth.** Swelling and tenderness in the region of

the bladder, with tensive and burning pain in the loins. *Violent pains* and *burning heat in the bladder.* * Very frequent micturition, with burning and cutting pains, so severe the patient screams aloud. Constant desire to urinate, with *scanty emissions of dark or bloody urine.* Abdomen distended and painful to contact.

**Caps.** Frequent but ineffectual desire to urinate. The urine is emitted in drops, is hot and burning. * Burning smarting in the urethra after micturition. The urine deposits a white sediment. * Shuddering and chilliness in the back.

**Caust.** Difficult, frequent, and painful micturition. The urine is light-colored, like water; it is loaded with lithic acid and lithates, with great debility. * Involuntary emissions of urine when coughing, or at night. Aching and crampy pains in the small of the back, in the region of the kidneys.

**Colch.** Persons of a gouty or rheumatic diathesis. Constant desire to urinate, with scanty emissions of *dark-red urine depositing a whitish sediment.* Burning and tenesmus in the urethra. Rheumatic pains in the limbs, especially during warm weather.

**Coni.** Especially old men, and persons suffering from excessive sexual indulgence. * The flow of urine suddenly stops, then continues at short intervals. Cutting pain in the urethra while urinating. Urine thick, white, and turbid. * Vertigo, particularly when lying down.

**Dig.** Inflammation of the neck of the bladder. Continual desire to urinate; each time only a few drops are emitted. * Frequent sharp, cutting pains in the neck of the bladder, as if a *straw was being thrust back and forth.* Urine dark brown and hot. Can retain the urine best in a recumbent posture.

**Dulc.** Painful pressing down in the region of the bladder. Urine turbid and white, or reddish and burning, depositing at times a red, at times a white sediment. * The disease was induced by exposure to damp, cold weather, or it gets worse every time the weather changes.

**Lachesis.** Dull pain in the bladder, and stitching pains in the region of the kidneys. Frequent micturition with copious discharge of foaming, dark urine. Yellow urine, the color of sulphur or saffron. *Sensation as if a ball were rolling in the bladder.* * Very unhappy and distressed after sleeping. Women at the climacteric period.

**Lyco.** Much pain in the small of the back, and pressure in the region of the kidneys. Stitches in the bladder and rectum. Pain in the back previous to urination, with relief as soon as the urine begins to flow. * *Red sediment like sand in the urine.* * Constant sense of fulness in the stomach. Cutting pain across the hypogastrium from right to left. * Great fear of being left alone.

**Merc.** Stinging pains in the small of the back, with a sensation of weakness. Constant desire to urinate, with scanty emissions of dark-red urine soon becoming turbid and fetid. The urine looks as if *mixed with blood*, with white flakes or as if containing pus. * Worse at night, and in damp rainy weather.

**Nux vom.** *Burning and lacerating pain in the neck of the bladder* and *urethra.* Painful, ineffectual desire to urinate, with discharge of a few drops of red, bloody, burning urine. Spasmodic stricture of the urethra, with retention of urine. * Constipation, with large, hard, difficult stools. Persons of sedentary or intemperate habits, or who suffer from hemorrhoids.

**Phos.** Contractive pain in the bladder, or stitches from the neck of the bladder to the anus. Urine white like curdled milk, soon becoming turbid with *brick-dust sediment.* Also brown urine, with sediment of red sand. Smarting, cutting, and jerking in the urethra. * Constipation, stools *long, narrow, hard,* and very difficult to expel.

**Phos. ac.** Great desire and urging to urinate, with pale face, heat and thirst. * Frequent micturition, the urine like milk mixed with jelly-like, bloody pieces, with pain in the kidneys. * Is very weak and indifferent to the affairs of life.

**Puls.** Aching, burning, and cutting pains in the region of the bladder. * Retention of urine, with redness, heat, and soreness of the vesical region externally. * Involuntary emissions of urine when sitting, coughing, or walking. * After urinating, spasmodic pain in the neck of the bladder, extending to the pelvis and thighs. *Scant, red, brown urine, with reddish, bloody, or mucous sediment.* Persons of a mild, tearful disposition.

**Rhus tox.** Involuntary emissions of urine at night or when at rest. Difficult urination, with drops of bloody urine. * Snow-white sediment in the urine. Rheumatic subjects; worse before a storm and in damp weather.

**Ruta g.** Frequent pressing to urinate, with scanty discharges of green urine. Pressure on the bladder as if continually full. * The pressure to urinate continues after micturition.

**Sarsa.** Tenesmus of the bladder, with cutting pain during micturition. Urine red, fiery, turbid, containing long flakes. The urine contains large quantities of pale sand. Children cry before and during micturition. Pain in the small of the back, extending towards the genital organs.

**Sulph.** Obstinate cases, the urine is mixed with mucus or blood; *very fetid.* * Burning in the urethra *during micturition.* Incontinence of urine, particularly at night. * Constant heat on top of the head. * Lank, lean persons who walk stooping.

**Terebinth.** Burning drawing pains in the kidneys. Pressure in the bladder extending up into the kidneys when sitting, disappearing when walking about. * Urine mixed with blood, forming a dirty reddish-brown or blackish fluid, with sediment like coffee-grounds.

---

## DELIRIUM TREMENS.

**Therapeutics.** Special indications.

**Arsen.** Pale, jaundiced complexion. Bloated face and cold blue skin. Fainting fits, particularly during vomiting. The patient imagines that vermin are crawling about the bed, and ugly animals are staring him in the face. * Great restlessness and fear of death. * Extreme thirst, drinks little and often.

**Bell.** Persons of a full *plethoric habit.* Flushed face and red eyes, with dilated pupils. * Boisterous delirium, with desire to escape. He tears the clothes, strikes, bites, and shrieks in his rage. * Sudden starting and jumping while sleeping.

**Camph.** Features distorted; eyes sunken; face, hands, and feet icy cold. Confusion of ideas, maniacal delirium, convulsions, frothing at the mouth, and insensibility. * Retention of urine, with constant pressure on the bladder.

**Coffea.** Headache as if a nail were driven into the brain. * Excessive irritability and wakefulness. Talks in his sleep and wakes with starting.

**Hyos.** Twitching and jerking of the muscles, especially of those about the eyes and face. *Furious delirium, with wild staring look,* dilated pupils, and throbbing of the carotids. Convulsive movements; subsultus tendinum. * Grasping at imaginary objects, muttering.

**Lachesis.** Where the throat is principally affected with difficult deglutition. * Cannot bear anything about the neck, not even his neck-tie. Talks much, flying from one subject to another. * The attacks are worse in the afternoon and after sleeping.

**Nux vom.** Trembling of the limbs and spasmodic twitching in different parts of the body. Incapable of thinking correctly. Makes frequent mistakes in talking. Delirium with frightful visions and efforts to escape. * Very irritable, and wishes to be alone. * Constipation with *large* difficult stools. Apprehensive of death.

**Opium.** Patient lies in a comatose state, with eyes half open. *Loud stertorous breathing.* * Complete loss of consciousness and sensation. * Delirious talking, with eyes wide open. Pupils widely dilated, or contracted. Pulse full and labored, or *slow and feeble.*

**Stram.** Disposed to talk continually. *Sings and prays most devoutly.* * Awakens with a shrinking look as if afraid of the first object seen. * Loquacious delirium, with desire to escape from bed. Dilatation of the pupils. Staring, somnolent eyes. Grinding of the teeth and distortions of the mouth.

The best remedies for the inclination to drink, and the evil effects of habitual drunkenness, are **Ars.**, **Nux vom.**, **Sulph.**, **Sulph. ac.**

---

## DENTITION.

**Therapeutics.** Special indications.

**Acon.** * Constant restlessness, which no change of position seems to relieve. The child cries, whines, or frets most of the time and cannot be quieted. * Dry, hot skin, disturbed sleep, much heat about the head, and *great thirst*. *Green watery diarrhœa*, or constipation.

**Apis m.** Frequent waking at night, or during sleep with screams. Red spots here and there over the whole body. Urine scanty, sometimes profuse. *Green-yellowish, watery diarrhœa*, worse in the morning. * Much yawning and uneasiness.

**Arsen.** The child has a very pale and waxen look, and is very weak. It often vomits all fluids soon after taking them, particularly water. * Drinks often, but little at a time. * Very restless, tossing from side to side. Fetid, undigested stools; dry and shrivelled skin.

**Bell.** The child moans a great deal; awakens from sleep in a fright, with staring eyes. * Starting and jumping during sleep. Face and eyes red, pupils dilated, head hot. * Convulsions, followed by sound sleep. Gums swollen and inflamed, with numerous *small blood-vessels showing on the surface.*

**Borax.** The child is very nervous, starts and jumps at the least noise. Sometimes it will start, cry out and hold on to things as if *afraid of falling.* * Cannot bear a downward motion even during sleep. * Aphthæ in the mouth, causing the child to cry out when nursing.

**Bryo.** Mouth and lips dry and parched. The child

wishes to be kept very quiet; gets faint and sick when raised up in bed. * The food is thrown up soon after taking it unchanged. Thirst for large draughts of water. * Hard, dry stools as if burnt, or morning diarrhœa. * Desire for things which are rejected when offered. Very irritable.

**Calc. c.** Large head with open fontanelles—scrofulous. Much perspiration about the head during sleep. * Cold damp feet. * White, chalk-like stools, or thin and whitish. Sour vomiting, or regurgitation of food. Swollen, distended abdomen, with emaciation and good appetite.

**Caust.** Children with delicate skin, which becomes chafed or excoriated during the process of teething. Prolonged constipation; *stools tough, covered with mucus, and shine like grease.* * Yellowish, sickly-looking face.

**Cham.** Great irritability and sensitiveness of the nervous system. Starting, uttering sudden cries and tossing about during sleep. * Very cross, wants to be carried all the time. * One cheek red and the other pale. Convulsive twitchings of the extremities. *Diarrhœa, with greenish, yellowish,* or *whitish, mucous stools, smelling like bad eggs.* Dry cough, especially during the night.

**Cicuta.** * Grinding of the teeth, with pressing of the jaws together, like lock-jaw. Convulsions, with limbs relaxed, hanging down, or stiff, rigid, and extended. A kind of half-sleep with tossing.

**Cina.** Paleness of the face, particularly around the nose and mouth. Disposition to pick or rub the nose. * Very restless during sleep, must be kept in motion all the time to be quieted. *Very peevish, wants many things which it rejects immediately.* * Urine whitish like milk. Grinding of the teeth; hacking cough.

**Coffea.** * The child is very excitable and sleepless. It *frets and worries in a pitiful manner*; cries one moment and laughs the next. The system is feverish, and the child is greatly exhausted for want of sleep.

**Cup. m.** Great uneasiness and tossing about. Convulsions, *beginning with cramps in the lower extremities and drawing in the fingers and toes;* much throwing about of the limbs, frothing at the mouth, and choking in the throat. Green painful stools and vomiting of mucus.

**Dulc.** Pale face, with circumscribed redness of the cheeks. Dry coryza and frequent sneezing. Diarrhœa with yellowish, greenish, or whitish stools. Nausea or real vomiting. * Symptoms all worse by every damp, cold change in the weather.

**Ferr.** Dentition advances very slowly, and an obstinate diarrhœa is the result. * Stools composed of mucus and undigested food. * Painless, exhausting diarrhœa, sometimes excoriating the parts. Vomiting of food soon after taking it. * Sudden flushing of the face. Emaciation, debility, and exhausting sweats.

**Graph.** *Unhealthy condition of the skin.* Rawness in the bends of the limbs, on the neck, and behind the ears. * Eruptions over the head and face which discharge a sticky, glutinous fluid. Constipation of large knotty stools.

**Hepar s.** Dry herpetic eruptions on the skin, especially in the bend of the arms, groin, upon the face and scalp, itching violently. * The gums are very tender and apparently very painful. Diarrhœa, stools whitish and smelling sour. Stomach inclined to be out of order; craves sour or strong-tasting things.

**Hyos.** The child continually puts its fingers into the mouth, presses its gums together as if chewing on something. Eyes red and sparkling. * Convulsions, beginning with twitching of the muscles of the face, especially about the eyes. Dark, bloated appearance of the face; dilated pupils. * Deep sleep, muttering, and picking at the bed-clothes. *Yellow, watery, involuntary stools.*

**Ignat.** Frequent flushes of heat, with perspiration. The child awakens from sleep with piercing cries, and trembling all over. Convulsive jerking of single parts. * The child is much distressed, *sighs, sobs*, and cries. Stools bloody mucous, often attended with tenesmus and prolapsus of the rectum.

**Ipecac.** Pale face, with blueness around the eyes. * Continual nausea, with frequent vomiting. Diarrhœa; stools green as grass, or fermented with many colors. Catarrh, with suffocative cough and rattling of mucus in the bronchia.

**Kreasote.** *Very painful dentition.* The protruding gum seems infiltrated with a dark, watery fluid. * The teeth begin to decay almost as soon as they are through the gums. The sufferings are usually *aggravated during the night.* Constipation, with hard, dry stools, or diarrhœa with dark-brown, watery, *very offensive stools.*

**Lach.** * The child always awakens in distress, and is worse after sleeping. Convulsions, which usually occur as the child goes to sleep Gums dark-purple and painful to touch. * Difficult deglutition, can't bear the throat to be touched.

**Lyco.** The child sleeps with its eyes partially closed, throwing its head from side to side, with moaning. Just before passing water, the child cries and screams as if in great pain. * Red sand-like sediment in the urine Much rumbling of wind in the bowels. Worse about four P. M., and better during the night.

**Mag. carb.** Green and sour-smelling diarrhœa which has continued a long time. * Stools green watery, resembling the scum of a frog-pond. Frequent vomiting of sour-smelling substances. Loss of appetite, emaciation.

**Merc.** * Copious salivation, redness of the gums, and sometimes little ulcers on the tongue and mouth. Diarrhœa, with greenish, slimy, or bloody stools, with *much straining.* Yellowish and strong-smelling urine. Aggravation at night.

**Nux vom.** The child is *very irritable* and cross. Loss of appetite with increased thirst. * Constipation, with large difficult stools, or small, frequent, lumpy, or brown mucous stools. * Especially suited to children raised on cow's - milk, &c., or whose mothers indulge in highly-seasoned food, wines, &c. Aggravation early in the morning.

**Nux mos.** Exhausting diarrhœa, with thin yellow stools, like beaten or stirred eggs. * The diarrhœa is accompanied with *great drowsiness.* Symptoms worse at night, and in warm weather.

**Podo. pel.** Restless sleep, with half-closed eyes;

moaning and grinding of the teeth. Rolling of the head from side to side. Green, watery, or whitish, chalk-like stools, very offensive, with frequent *gagging or empty retching*. * Morning diarrhœa, with prolapsus ani during every stool. Aggravation in hot weather, and after eating and drinking.

**Rheum.** When during dentition a *sour-smelling diarrhœa* is developed, with *colic before and tenesmus after stool.* * Sour smell of the whole body, which washing does not remove. Diarrhœa worse by moving about, or from uncovering any part of the body.

**Silicea.** * Large head with open fontanelles—*scrofulous.* Profuse sour-smelling perspiration on the head. Hard, hot, distended abdomen. The protruding gum seems blistered, and is very sensitive. * Constipation, the stool suddenly *recedes after having been partially expelled.*

**Stram.** The child's brain seems to be much disturbed. Violent grinding of the teeth. Moving of the fingers during sleep as if searching for something. * Convulsions, with cries as if frightened by the sight of hideous objects. Agitation of the limbs, particularly of the arms and hands, *with motions of the fingers.* * Thin, blackish stools, having a putrid smell.

**Sulph.** Face pale or sallow. *Open fontanelles.* * Eruptions on the skin attended with much itching. Restless nights, with frequent waking. Diarrhœa, with whitish, greenish, or bloody mucous stools, and excoriation of the anus. * Early morning diarrhœa. Frequent vomiting of the food taken. * Frequent weak, faint spells.

**Sulph. ac.** *Aphthæ of the mouth and gums,* with much slavering. The child is very irritable, and cries much of the time. * Diarrhœa, the stools look like chopped, saffron-yellow mucus. Loss of appetite, and *great debility.*

**Verat. alb.** Vomiting, and severe empty retching, aggravated by the least motion. * Diarrhœa, each stool followed by great prostration and cold sweat on the forehead. Cold damp feeling of the extremities. * Very weak, faint pulse. * Violent thirst for large quantities of cold water.

## DIARRHŒA.

**Therapeutics.** Special indications.

**Acon.** Stools frequent and scanty, *watery, whitish, or slimy.* Nausea and sweat *before,* and *tenesmus during* stool. General dry heat, full and frequent pulse. * Vertigo or fainting on rising up. Restlessness and intense thirst. * If caused by checked perspiration, or exposure to a cold dry wind.

**Aloes.** Stools *yellow fecal, copious and watery.* Is driven out of bed early every morning to stool. *Before* stool, a feeling of weight and fulness in the pelvis. *During* stool, tenesmus and heat in the rectum and anus. Prominent hemorrhoids, tender to touch. * Loud gurgling in the abdomen as of water running out of a bottle. Diarrhœa *worse after eating.*

**Ant. c.** Stools *watery* and profuse, with *deranged stomach.* * Tongue coated white. *Violent vomiting of bitter, bilious,* or *slimy mucus ; worse after eating or drinking.* If caused by overloading the stomach.

**Apis.** Stools *greenish, yellowish, slimy mucous,* or *yellow watery.* * Sensation in the abdomen as if something would break, when straining at stool. Tongue dry and shining; little or no thirst. Œdema of the feet. Aggravation in the morning.

**Argen. nit.** Stools *green, fetid mucous,* passing off with much flatus. *Nausea with loud eructations.* Vomiting of glassy, tenacious mucus. Aggravation at night, after midnight, and after eating sweet things.

**Arnica.** Stools *slimy mucous,* or brown fermented (like yeast). Bitter or putrid taste in the mouth. * Putrid eructations, as if from rotten eggs. *Aversion to food; bad breath.* If caused by mechanical injuries.

**Arsen.** Stools *thick, dark green mucous, or brown, black, and watery.* During stool, tenesmus, burning in the anus and rectum. * Great weakness, fainting, and rapid exhaustion. * Restlessness, constantly changing from side to side. * Great thirst, drinking often but little at a time. *Vomiting after eating or drinking.* Aggravation at night, after midnight, after eating or drinking.

**Bell.** Stools *thin*, *green mucous*, or white watery mucous, small and frequent. Clutching pains in the abdomen. * Pains which come on suddenly and cease as suddenly. * Sleepy, but cannot sleep. * Sudden starting and jumping during sleep. Throbbing headache. Aggravation in the afternoon, and after sleeping.

**Benz. ac.** Stools *watery* or *light-colored; copious; very offensive.* * Strong-smelling urine, mostly dark-colored. Feels weak and exhausted.

**Bry.** Diarrhœa in *hot weather*, or when the disease was induced by *taking cold drinks* when the *system was heated.* Stools brown, thin fecal, or undigested. * Nausea and faintness from sitting up. * Thirst for large quantities of water, at long intervals. Aggravation *in the morning; from motion;* after suppressed exanthemata.

**Calc. c.** Diarrhœa of scrofulous persons. Swollen, distended abdomen, with emaciation and good appetite. Stools *whitish or watery. Chronic diarrhœa*, with clay like stools. * Profuse sweat on the head when sleeping. * Feet cold as if they had on damp stockings. Difficult urination; urine clear, smelling strong and fetid.

**Carb. veg.** Stools *light-colored; involuntary; putrid; cadaverous-smelling.* Mostly in the last stage, and where the vital powers are greatly exhausted. * Emissions of large quantities of flatus, inodorous or putrid. *Restlessness and anxiety.* Aggravation from 5 to 6 P. M.

**Cham.** Stools *green, watery, corroding, with colic.* * Hot diarrhœic stools smelling like bad eggs. Bitter taste with bilious vomiting. * Very impatient, can hardly answer one civilly. * Children are very cross and fretful, and must be carried all the time. * One cheek red and the other pale. Aggravation at night, and during dentition.

**China.** Stools *yellowish, watery, whitish*, or *blackish*, with severe spasmodic colic relieved by bending double. *Painless, undigested*, offensive stools, with much distention of the abdomen. * Great weakness and inclination to sweat. *Emissions of large quantities of fetid flatus.* Thirst, drinks often, but little at a time. Aggravation *at night*, after eating, and *every other day.*

**Cina.** *White, papescent stools.* Paleness of the face, particularly around the nose and mouth. * Disposition to pick and bore at the nose. * White, turbid, or jelly-like urine. *Restless sleep, frequently changing position,* and waking with cries. Grinding of the teeth during sleep. Adapted to persons troubled with worms.

**Colo.** Stools *saffron-yellow, frothy, or thin, slimy, and watery.* Before stool cutting colic, great urging. * Feeling in the abdomen as if the intestines were being squeezed between stones. Severe colicky pains mostly around the navel, relieved by bending double. Great thirst; bitter taste in the mouth. Aggravation after taking the least nourishment.

**Crot. tig.** * Stools *yellow, watery,* or greenish-yellow, *expelled with great force.* Aggravation after *drinking, while eating.* Gagging with vertigo, worse after drinking. Colic and writhing around the umbilicus.

**Dulc.** Stools yellowish, greenish, watery or whitish. Colic before and during stool. Griping pain in the region of the navel, with vomiting of mucus. * If the disease was caused by taking cold, or is aggravated in cold damp weather. *Dry heat of the skin.*

**Ferrum.** Painless diarrhœa. Stools *copious, watery, undigested.* Bowels feel sore as if bruised. Emaciation, debility, good appetite. Vomiting of the food soon after eating it. * The least emotion or exertion produces a red flushed face.

**Gels.** Diarrhœa induced by *sudden depressing emotions, fright, grief, bad news.* Stools the color of tea, dark-yellow. Desire to be quiet. Little or no thirst.

**Gum. gutt.** Stools *yellow* or *green, mixed with mucus; very offensive.* Before and during stool, strong urging, with hot pinching pain in the abdomen. * Feeling of great relief after stool, as if an irritating substance were removed from the intestines. * *Rapid expulsion of the stool.*

**Hepar.** Painless or *chronic* diarrhœa. Stools *light-yellow, green, slimy, undigested.* * Sour-smelling diarrhœa. Better after eating. Hot, sour regurgitation of food. * Feeling of fulness in the stomach, with desire to loosen the clothing.

**Hell. nig.** * White, jelly-like mucous stools, with rging and tenesmus. In protracted and dangerous ases, during dentition, or acute hydrocephalus. *omiting of green or blackish* substances.

**Hyos.** *Painless, yellow watery diarrhœa.* * Involntary stools without being conscious of it. Diarrhœa uring typhoid fever, and in lying-in women.

**Ipec.** Stools *grass-green mucous; fermented.* Before nd during stool, nausea and colic. * Vomiting of ellow, green, or jelly-like mucus. Paleness of the ace, and coldness of the extremities. * *Flatulent colic,* ith pinching, griping about the umbilicus.

**Iris vers.** Painful, green, watery stools, worse at ight, about two or three o'clock A. M. * Burning in he rectum and anus after stool. Periodical diarrhœa. omiting of *sour fluid, with burning in the mouth and auces.*

**Iodine.** Especially in *chronic* diarrhœa. Stools *atery, foaming, whitish.* Patient feels better after eatng. * Restlessness, continually changing position. maciation with good appetite. Scrofulous persons.

**Kali c.** Chronic diarrhœa, with *light, gray, fecal tools,* followed by burning in the anus. Painless liarrhœa with much rumbling in the abdomen. * Little sac-like swellings on the upper eyelids in the norning.

**Lep. vir.** * Stools *black, papescent, tar-like, very fetid.* After stool, sharp cutting pains and distress in he umbilical region. Aggravation in the afternoon r evening. After exposure to wet, damp weather.

**Lyco.** Chronic diarrhœa. Stools thin, brown, pale, fetid. A feeling of great fulness in the stomach after eating but little. Pain and tenderness of the stomach, relieved by loosening the clothing. * Red sediment like sand in the urine. In weak dyspeptic persons. * Aggravation about 4 P. M., and in the morning.

**Mag. carb.** *Sour-smelling* diarrhœa of children. * Stools resembling the scum of a frog-pond, or green, slimy, and watery. Before stool, cutting and pinching pain in the abdomen. *Sour vomiting.* Œdema of the feet up to the calves.

**Merc.** Stools *dark-green, slimy, frothy,* or *bloody* * Frequent urging and *tenesmus,* during and *after* stool Cutting, pinching pain in the abdomen, with chilliness. Bitter bilious vomiting. Violent thirst for cold drinks. Aphthæ in the mouth, and increased flow of saliva. *Sour-smelling night-sweat, particularly about the head, cold on the forehead.* Worse at night and in hot weather.

**Nux mos.** Stools *thin yellow, like stirred eggs.* Before stool, cutting pain in the abdomen. * Loss of appetite, and *great drowsiness.* Colic worse after eating or drinking. The *tongue is very dry,* it sticks to the mouth. Great distention of the abdomen after every meal. Worse at night and in cool damp weather

**Nux vom.** Frequent small *watery, slimy, brownish mucous* stools. Colic and tenesmus before and during stool, with *relief after.* Dysenteric diarrhœa. * Symptoms *worse early in* the morning. * Nausea and sour bitter vomiting. After the use of quack nostrums and for persons of intemperate habits.

**Phos.** Chronic *painless* diarrhœa, worse in the morning. Stools *undigested, watery, with little white flakes* or *lumps like sago.* Gradual loss of strength. Thirst for very cold drinks. * Vomiting of what has been drunk as soon as it becomes warm in the stomach. *Sleepy in the daytime, particularly after meals.*

**Phos. ac.** *Painless* diarrhœa. Stools *whitish-watery,* or yellowish and very offensive. The diarrhœa is accompanied with great rumbling in the bowels. * Very indifferent, wants nothing, and cares for nothing. Frequent *emissions* of *pale, watery urine.* Profuse perspiration at night.

**Podo. pel.** Painless diarrhœa. *Profuse watery stools,* with meal-like sediment; also yellow mucous stools *smelling like carrion. Before* stool, loud gurgling in the bowels as of water. * *During* stool, prolapsus ani. Gagging or empty retching. Cramp in the feet, calves, and thighs. * Always *worse in the morning,* at night, and in hot weather.

**Puls.** Stools *greenish, yellowish, like bile.* * Very changeable stools, no two alike. Before stool, rumbling and cutting pain in the bowels. * Diarrhœa,

*›orse at night*, from eating fruit, or ice-cream. Bitter ıste in the mouth after eating. * Craves cool fresh ir, worse in a close, warm room. Inclination to be hilly even in a warm room. White-coated tongue; ›ss of taste; thirstlessness.

**Rheum.** Stools *green, brown, fermented, smelling ›ur.* Colic *before* and *during* stool, and *tenesmus* after. The whole body has a *sour smell*, which cannot be emoved by washing. Cutting colic, relieved by bendıg double. Diarrhœa during dentition.

**Rhus tox.** Stools *reddish mucous*, or *yellowish mu›us.* Cutting colic *before* and *during* stool, with relief *fter* stool. Troublesome dreams. Involuntary stools t night while sleeping. * Aggravation at night, and ›hen *at rest.*

**Secale.** Painless diarrhœa. Stools *brown, watery,* r *slimy; discharged rapidly and with great force.* Great xhaustion during and after stool. Vomiting without ffort, with great weakness. Great anxiety, and burnıg at the pit of the stomach. * *Aversion to heat*, or *to eing covered up.* Extreme thirst.

**Sulph.** Stools very changeable, *yellow, brown, reen, undigested. Early morning diarrhœa*, driving the atient out of bed in a hurry. Before stool, urging nd cutting colic. * Constant heat on top of the head. our or bitter vomiting. * Frequent, weak, faint pells. Drowsiness during the day, and wakeful at ight. *After suppressed eruptions.*

**Sulph. ac.** Diarrhœa with great debility. Pain›ss, chronic diarrhœa. Stools *saffron-colored mucous, ›ringy, green, watery.* Coldness and relaxed feeling in ıe stomach. Sour eructations. * Sensation of tremor ll over the body without trembling. Aphthæ in the ıouth.

**Thuya.** Copious, *pale-yellow, watery stools, discharged ›ith great force; gurgling like water from a bung-hole.* ›apid exhaustion and emaciation. Aggravation in ıe morning, after breakfast and after drinking coffee.

**Verat. alb.** Stools *profuse watery, blackish* or *green›h.* Severe pinching colic *before* and during stool. After stool, *great weakness* and empty feeling in the bdomen. * The suffering causes a cold sweat to stand on the forehead. Violent vomiting of frotl mucus. * Violent thirst for large quantities of co water. *Excessive weakness.*

---

## DIPHTHERIA.

**Therapeutics.** Special indications.

**Acon.** In the forming stage. Dry, hot skin, ar very quick pulse. Dark redness of the fauces, velu palati, and tonsils. Burning, fine piercing sensatic in the throat. * Great fear and anxiety of mind, wi nervous excitability. * Very sensitive to contact.

**Apis m.** Great debility from the beginning. Tl membrane assumes at once a dirty-grayish colo Puffiness around the eyes, and pain in the ears whe swallowing. * Stinging pains in the affected part Itching stinging eruption on the skin. Numbness c the feet and hands.

**Arsen.** Great anguish, extreme restlessness ar fear of death. Fetid breath, and viscid foul discharg from the nostrils. * Constant desire for cold drink but can take but little at a time. * Great and increa ing prostration. All worse about midnight.

**Arum tri.** Throat raw and sore, as if excoriate Putrid odor from the mouth. * Burning, *ichoro discharge from the nose, excoriating the nostrils and upp lip.* Cracked corners of the mouth and lips. Sul maxillary glands swollen. Urine abundant and pale

**Bell.** Great dryness of the fauces; tonsils brigh red and swollen. Cannot swallow, or only with th greatest difficulty. * Very restless, feels drowsy y cannot sleep. * Starts in his sleep, or jumps su denly up in bed. Congestion to the head, with throl bing of the carotid arteries; eyes injected; delirium

**Bromine.** The disease commences in the laryn and rises up into the fauces. In some cases it exten into the larynx, producing a croupy cough and muc rattling of mucus. * Suffocating cough, with hoars whistling, croupy sound.

**Bry.** Formation of false membrane on the tonsils and palate. Lips parched, dry, and cracked. Thirst for large draughts of water. * Wants to remain perfectly still, as the least motion increases his suffering. Cannot sit up on account of nausea and faintness. * Hard, dry stools as if burnt.

**Calc. chlor.** This remedy (Chloride of Lime) is highly commended by Dr. Neidhard in all stages of the disease. He says, it not only cured the ordinary diphtheria, but the most dangerous cases, and also diphtheric croup. He uses it both in trituration and in solution.

**Canth.** Burning and dryness in the mouth, extending to the throat and pharynx. Extreme prostration, sinking, death-like turns. * Constant desire to urinate, passing but a few drops at a time.

**Cap. an.** Burning and soreness in the mouth and throat. Congested appearance of the mucous membrane. Fauces partially covered with the diphtheric deposit. Heat and throbbing in the head. Rapid pulse, vertigo and bleeding at the nose. * Chilliness in the back.

**Kali bi.** Fauces inflamed, and more or less covered with a dirty-yellow deposit forming pseudo-membrane. * Hoarse croupy cough, with expectoration of *stringy* mucus. Deep-eating ulcers in the fauces. Tough stringy discharge from the nose. Swelling of the parotid glands.

**Lachesis.** The disease mostly appears on the *left* side first. Throat greatly swollen internally and externally. Discharge from the nose and mouth of a very fetid and excoriating fluid. * Can bear nothing to touch the larynx and throat, — it is so painful. *Fauces covered with a diphtheric membrane.* * Patient worse after sleeping.

**Lyco.** * The disease commences on the *right* side of the throat and spreads to the left. Brownish-red appearance of the fauces. Stitching pains in the throat when swallowing. Nose stopped up, and the patient cannot breathe with the mouth shut. * Widely dilated nostrils with every inspiration. Awakens from sleep very cross and irritable. * Red sand in the urine.

**Merc. iod.** * Pseudo-membranous deposit upon the tonsils, uvula, velum palati, and pharynx. Tongue coated with a thick, yellow, dirty coating. Tonsils much swollen, and there is great difficulty in swallowing. * Breath very offensive. *Expectoration of much tough fetid saliva.* Hoarse breathing. Swelling of the parotid and submaxillary glands.

**Nitric ac.** Spreading ulcers in the mouth and throat. Putrid-smelling breath. Swelling of the submaxillary and parotid glands. Corroding discharge from the nose. Dry, barking cough; intermittent pulse. * Strong-smelling urine, like that of horses. * Sore throat, extending up into the nose, with profuse, thin purulent discharge.

**Phytolacca.** * Fauces, tonsils, and pharynx covered with dark-colored pseudo-membrane. Excessive fetor of the breath. Great prostration, is unable to stand. When rising up in bed, gets faint and dizzy. Violent aching in the back and limbs.

---

## DYSENTERY.

**Therapeutics.** Special indications.

**Acon.** Usually in the beginning of the disease. Stools frequent, small, bloody, or slimy mucous. During stool cutting pains and tenesmus. * Vertigo on rising up. General dry heat and *great restlessness.* * Fear of death; predicts the day he will die.

**Aloes.** Stools *bloody, jelly-like mucous. Before* stool, a sense of fulness and weight in the pelvis, and pain around the navel. *During* stool, *tenesmus and burning in the rectum.* * Loud gurgling in the bowels, like water running out of a bottle. Large and prominent hemorrhoids, tender to touch.

**Arnica.** Dysentery caused by mechanical injuries. Stools *clear mucous,* or *bloody, with tenesmus.* Bitter or putrid taste in the mouth. * Putrid eructations as if from bad eggs.

**Arsen.** Stools *dark or blackish fluid, mixed with*

*ood, of a putrid foul smell. During* stool, tenesmus nd burning in the rectum. * Great anguish, rest-ssness, and fear of death. * Extreme thirst, drinks ften, but little at a time. Rapid prostration and sink-ng of the vital forces. Aggravation at *night*, or *after ating* or *drinking.*

**Baptisia.** Stools *scant, bloody mucous. Before* and uring stool, violent colicky pains in the hypogastri-m. During stool great tenesmus. * Soreness of the esh and whole body, with chilliness. * The sweat, rine, and stools, are all extremely fetid.

**Belladon.** Stools *greenish, slimy, bloody.* Great *enesmus during* and *after* stool. * Clutching pains in he abdomen, which appear suddenly, and cease as uddenly. * Pains are relieved by stopping the breath nd bearing down. Abdomen hot and tender to pres-ure. Sleepiness with restless tossing about. * Sud-len starting, and jumping during sleep. *Mouth and hroat very dry, with little or no thirst.*

**Bryonia.** The disease was induced by getting overheated, or from taking cold drinks when the sys-em was very warm. *Thin bloody stools,* preceded by utting colic. * Sitting up in bed causes nausea and omiting. * The patient wants to keep very still. Thirst for large quantities of water at long intervals. Aggravation in the morning and by motion.

**Cantharis.** Stools *white or pale-reddish, like scrapings of the intestines.* Great tenesmus and burning, sting-ng in the anus. * Frequent urging to urinate, with slight and painful discharge. High fever, with burn-ng and dryness of the mouth, *burning thirst,* or *no thirst at all.*

**Caps.** Stools bloody mucous, or mucous streaked with black blood. * After stool, tenesmus and thirst, with shuddering after drinking. Tenesmus of the bladder. Distention of the abdomen as if it would burst. * Chilliness in the back. * Taste as of putrid water in the mouth.

**Carb. veg.** Mostly in advanced stages. Stools of *foul blood and mucus; involuntary, smelling terribly.* * Great prostration, and cold breath. * The patient wants more air and to be fanned all the time. Heat about the head, and cold perspiration on the ex tremities.

**Cham.** Stools frequent, *small, green* or *white mu cous,* smelling like bad eggs. Colic before and durin stool. * Very impatient, can hardly answer on civilly. * Children are very fretful, must be carrie all the time to be appeased. * One cheek red and ho and the other pale and cold. In the first stages, an during dentition.

**China.** Weakly persons, and others who have los much blood. Stools *chocolate-colored, smelling putric Before* stool colic, relieved by bending double. Aggra vation at night, and after a meal. Great weaknes and inclination to sweat. * Patient worse ever other day.

**Colch.** Stools *jelly-like mucous,* or *bloody, mingle with a skinny substance,* attended with *severe colic an tenesmus.* During stool, spasms of the sphincter ani with a shuddering over the back. * Autumnal dysen tery, when the days are warm and the nights cool Œdema of the lower extremities; urine dark-brow and scant.

**Colocynth.** Stools *bloody mucous. Before* stool cutting pain and great urging. * *Violent colicky pains mostly around the navel, causing the patient to bend double* Relief after every evacuation. Abdomen distende and painful to contact. Patient worse after a meal.

**Dulc.** Stools *green mucous, or bloody.* If the dis ease was induced by exposure to cold. * Symptom all aggravated by every cold change in the weather Dry heat of the skin, and much thirst.

**Ipecac.** Stools *bloody,* or *bloody mucous.* Grea pressing to stool, with griping and pinching about th navel. * Much nausea and vomiting. Disgust an loathing of all kinds of food. If caused by eating un ripe, sour fruit. No thirst.

**Kali bi.** Stools bloody, or jelly-like. *Durin* stool, painful urging and tenesmus. Gnawing pai about the navel. * Tongue dry, smooth, red, an cracked. Much thirst, desire for acids. Aggravatio in the morning.

**Mag. car.** Stools *bloody mucous,* or *green slimy mu*

*us.* *Before* stool cutting and pinching in the abdoien. *During* and *after* stool *tenesmus.* Tongue coated irty-yellow. Sour vomiting. In children during entition.

**Merc. cor.** Stools *pure blood,* or *bloody mucus.* *)uring* stool, painful pressing, straining, and tenesius. Almost constant cutting pain in the abdomen, iostly around the umbilicus. * *Great tenesmus* of the *ladder,* with scanty secretion of urine.

**Merc. sol.** Stools *bloody mucous,* or *green, slimy.* *3efore* stool, violent and frequent urging. *During* and *fter* stool, *violent tenesmus.* * Wants to remain a long ime at the chamber. Pinching and cutting colic, with hilliness and shuddering. Prolapsus ani. Violent hirst for cold drinks. Profuse night sweats, particuarly on the head. All the symptoms worse at night, nd in damp rainy weather.

**Nitric ac.** Stools profuse, bloody. *Before* stool, rawing colicky pain. *During* stool, *tenesmus* and pasmodic contraction of the anus. Long-lasting pains, which are very exhausting. * Spreading ulcers in the nouth, with fetid breath.

**Nux vom.** Stools *thin, bloody mucous,* sometimes ningled with *hard lumps* of *fæcal matter.* *Before* stool, onstant urging; back-ache as if broken. *During* tool, violent tenesmus, and cutting pain in the hypogastrium, with desire to vomit. *After* stool, relief. * Persons of intemperate habits, or who have been lrugged with nostrums. *Symptoms worse in the morning.* * Patient very irritable, and wants to be alone.

**Phos.** Stools green, slimy, or bloody. Painless lysentery. The anus remains open as if paralyzed. Symptoms *worse in the morning, and from lying on the left side.* Thirst for very cold drinks, which are thrown up as soon as they get warm in the stomach.

**Podo. pel.** Stools *bloody and green mucous,* or *jelly-like mucous.* Disease attended with little or no pain. *Prolapsus ani* during and after stool. Children *toss their heads from side to side.* * Gagging or empty retching. Aggravation in the morning, at night, and during dentition. Loud rumbling in the bowels.

**Puls.** Stools blood-streaked mucous. *Before* stool,

rumbling and cutting colic. During stool, chilline and pain in the back. Thick yellow coat on th tongue. Bitter taste in the mouth. * Thirstlessnes * Worse towards evening and at night.

**Rhus tox.** Stools reddish mucous, or jelly-lik *Before* and *during* stool, cutting colic. * Pain whic runs in streaks down the limbs with every evacuatior *Remission of the pains after stool, and from moving abou*

**Staph.** Stools, yellow mucous. *Before* and afte stool, cutting pains in the bowels. During stool, *tene mus* of *the rectum and bladder.* Always worse afte drinking cold water.

**Sulph.** Stools green mucous, or blood-streake mucous; changeable. *Before* stool cutting coli After stool tenesmus. *Painful sensitiveness of the abdo men, as if the internal parts were raw and sore.* * Weak faint spells, frequently through the day. Dysentery consequent upon suppressed cutaneous eruption * Lean persons, who walk stooping, or who suffer fro piles.

---

## DYSMENORRHŒA.

**Therapeutics.** Special indications.

**Ammo. c.** Menses premature and abundant, pre ceded by griping colic and loss of appetite. Discharg blackish, in clots, passing off with pain in the abdo men. Paleness of the face, sadness, and toothache.

**Bell.** The pains precede the flow, with congestion t the head and confusion of sight. Frightful vision and screaming. * Disposition to bite and tear things Redness and bloatedness of the face. * Strong *bearin down* in the lower parts of the abdomen, as if every thing would escape through the vulva. * Pains com on suddenly and cease just as suddenly. Discharg copious, and of a bright-red color; sometimes clotte and offensive.

**Cactus.** Menses scanty and cease flowing whe lying down. * Terrible pains causing her to cr t aloud and weep. Pains come on periodically, ıstly in the evening. * A feeling as if the heart was ıstricted with an iron band. Palpitation of the art, worse when lying on the left side.

**Calc. c.** Preceding the flow, swelling and tender-ss of the breasts, headache, colic, shiverings and ıcorrhœa. During the flow, cutting in the abdomen, othache, bearing down in the abdomen, and enlarge-ınt of the veins. * Feet cold as if they had on mp stockings. *Scrofulous diathesis.*

**Cham.** Pressure towards the uterus, resembling *ıor-pains.* * Discharge dark-colored and coagu-ed, with tearing pains in the thighs. Frequent de-e to pass urine. Bloated red face, or *one cheek red d the other pale.* Hot perspiration about the head. Very impatient, can hardly answer one civilly.

**Cimicifu.** Scanty or profuse flow of coagulated ood. * Severe pains in the back, down the thighs d through the hips. Labor-like pains with heavy essing down. Hysteric spasms, cramps, tenderness the hypogastric region. Low-spirited and very nsitive.

**Conium.** Discharge scant, and brown in appear-ce. Previous to the menses, the breasts swell, be-me hard and painful. Pressing downwards in the ıdomen and drawing in the legs. * Much difficulty voiding urine, it stops and starts repeatedly. Aching pains about the heart, and vertigo when ing down or turning over in bed. Painful abdomi-l spasms.

**Nux vom.** Menses return too soon, discharge ick and clotted. Writhing pains in the abdomen with ıusea, or pain in the back and loins as if dislocated. Soreness across the pubis as if bruised. Frequent sire to pass urine. Constipation with frequent urg-g, hard difficult stools. After the use of drugs ıd nostrums.

**Phos.** Menses too early and scant. Very sleepy ıring the flow, she can hardly keep awake. Stitches the mammæ, sour eructations and vomiting of sour ıbstances. Great fermentation in the abdomen. ıtting in the hypogastric region, chilliness, cold hands and feet. * Sensation of weakness and emp ness in the abdomen. * *Long, narrow,* hard stoo very difficult to expel.

**Puls.** Delayed menses, the blood is thick a black, flowing by fits and starts. Feeling of heavin as if from a stone in the pelvic cavity. * Pains violent that she tosses about in all directions, wi cries and tears. Drawing sensation and numbn extending down the thighs. * Vertigo on rising u with chilliness. * Mild, tearful woman. *Worse in warm room.*

**Sepia.** Menses too early and scant. Colicky pai and *great bearing down, obliging her to cross the lim* Before the menses, leucorrhœa, excoriating the par * Painful sensation of emptiness at the pit of t stomach. Sick stomach, particularly in the mornin Constipation of hard, knotty, difficult stools, with sensation of *weight in the anus.*

**Sulph.** Discharge thick, black, and acrid. Vi lent pinching in the abdomen, with great heat, chil ness, and sort of epilepsy. * Constant heat in top the head. * Frequent flashes of heat and weak fai spells. Chronic cutaneous eruptions. *Lean perso who walk stooping.*

---

## DYSPEPSIA.

**Therapeutics.** Special indications.

**Ant. cr.** The disease was caused by overloadi the stomach. Tongue *coated white.* * Eructatio tasting of the food last eaten. Nausea and vomitin Watery stools, mingled with hard lumps. *Thirst, wo at night.*

**Arnica.** If caused by a blow or concussion. So bruised feeling in the stomach. Eructations, tasti like bad eggs. Sense of fulness in the pit of t stomach. Tongue coated yellow. After meals, inc nation to vomit. Bitter or putrid taste.

**Arsen.** Derangement of the stomach from ic

cream, fruit, and acid things. * Nausea and vomiting after eating or drinking. Heat or *burning in the stomach.* * Intense thirst, drinking often but little at a time. Anxious restlessness. *Rapid prostration of strength.* * Pressure as of a stone in the stomach.

**Bry.** Dyspepsia occurring in hot weather, or from drinking cold water when over-heated. Loathing of food, sometimes so violent that even the smell of it is intolerable. Stitching pains in the stomach, worse from motion or pressure. Soreness over the region of the stomach. *Frequent eructations, especially after a meal.* Food is thrown up immediately after eating. * Constipation, stools dry and hard as if burnt. * Is very irritable, everything vexes him.

**Calc. c.** Pressure as of a weight in the stomach. * Cannot bear anything tight around the hypochondrium. Sour taste in the mouth. Vomiting of the ingesta, which tastes sour. Aversion to meat and warm food, with desire for dainties. * Cold damp feet. *Profuse menstruation.* Cannot sleep after 3 A. M. Stools large, hard, and sometimes only partially digested.

**Carb. v.** Frequent eructations affording only temporary relief. The most innocent kind of food disagrees with the stomach. * Sensation as if the stomach and abdomen would burst when eating or drinking. Sour rancid belchings, and burning in the stomach. After debauching.

**Cham.** Painful bloatedness of the epigastrium in the morning, with a sensation as if the contents were rising to the chest. * Aching pain in the stomach and under the short ribs. Bitter taste with bilious vomiting. * Very impatient, can hardly answer a civil question.

**China.** * Abdomen feels full and tight as if stuffed, eructations affording no relief. * Aversion to every kind of nourishment. Craves wine or sour things. Eructations tasting of the ingesta. Debility with desire to lie down *after every meal.* Weakly persons who have lost much blood.

**Gel. sem.** Feeling of emptiness and weakness in the stomach and bowels. Distention of the stomach with pain and nausea. Burning in the stomach extending up to the mouth. * Symptoms all worse from sudden emotions, fright, grief, or bad news. * False hunger — a kind of gnawing in the stomach.

**Hepar.** The stomach is easily disordered despite the utmost care. Craving for acids or strong acrid articles. Nausea, and eructations without taste or smell. Putrid or metallic taste. * Accumulation of mucus in the throat. Hard, difficult stools. Risings in the œsophagus as if he had been eating sour things.

**Hydras.** * Dull aching pain in the stomach, which causes a very weak faint feeling. Burning pain in the umbilical region. Eructations of sour fluid. Cutting pain in the stomach. * A feeling of goneness in the region of the stomach, with violent palpitation of the heart.

**Lyc.** Feeling of great fulness and heaviness in the stomach after a meal. * After taking a mere swallow of food, feels full up to the throat. * Constant sense of fermentation in the abdomen, like yeast working. *Much rumbling, particularly in the left hypochondria.* Distressing pain in the back before urinating. * Red sand in the urine. Constipation, stools hard, scant, and passed with great difficulty. Symptoms worse about 4 P. M.

**Merc.** * Very sensitive about the pit of the stomach and abdomen. When sitting, the food feels like a stone in the stomach. *Pressure in the epigastrium,* eructations and heartburn after a meal. Aversion to solid food, meat, warm food, with desire for refreshing things. Much salivation, with saltish, metallic taste.

**Nux vom.** Putrid or bitter taste in the mouth early in the morning. *Frequent sour eructations.* * Region of the stomach is very sensitive to pressure. *Cramp-like pains in the stomach, with pressure, particularly after a meal.* Cannot bear the clothing fastened. * Rising of sour and bitter fluids from the stomach. * Very irritable, and wishes to be alone. Constipation with frequent urging, and a sensation as if the anus were contracted. Persons of sedentary or intemperate habits, or the victims of drugs and nostrums

**Puls.** Tongue *coated white* or *yellow, with bad taste in the morning.* * Eructations after a meal, tasting of the food last eaten. *Beating in the region of the stomach.* All kinds of fatty food, pork, pastry, ice-cream, etc., particularly disagree. * Vertigo when stooping or rising from a sitting posture. Chilliness and flashes of heat. *No thirst.* Nightly diarrhœa. Mild, tearful disposition.

**Sepia.** Pulsations in the stomach during a meal. * Great weakness of digestion. Sour or bitter eructations. Pressure on the stomach as of a stone. * Yellowness of the face, with a streak across the nose resembling a saddle. * Constipation of hard, knotty, difficult stools, with a sense of weight in the anus.

**Silicea.** Bitter taste in the morning. Nausea, especially in the morning, or after a meal. * Water tastes badly; vomits after drinking. Pains in the stomach with water-brash. No appetite, but great thirst. * Constipation, the *stool recedes after having been partly expelled.*

**Staph.** Sensation as if the stomach were hanging down relaxed. Soon after full and substantial meal the patient feels hungry. * Extreme hunger, even when the stomach is full of food.

**Sulph.** Sour eructations and much troublesome acidity in the stomach. Region of the stomach sensitive to contact. Feels very weak and faint about 11 A. M.; must have something to eat. * Frequent weak faint spells. * Burning heat on top of the head. * Early morning diarrhœa. * Lean persons who walk stooping.

---

## ENCEPHALITIS.

**Therapeutics.** Special indications.

**Acon.** In the commencement, when there is a high degree of fever, evinced by a *hot, dry* skin and hard, quick pulse. Congestion of blood to the head, with redness of the face. * Great anxiety and fear of death, predicts the day he will die. * Sleeplessness, restlessness, tossing from side to side. Vertigo or fainting on rising up.

**Bell.** Violent throbbing and stitching pains in the head. * Red sparkling eyes, with furious look. *Face red and bloated.* Great heat in the head, with violent throbbing of the carotids. * Furious delirium, with desire to escape from bed; he tries to strike, bite, and injure those around him. * Great intolerance of noise and light. Pupils contracted or dilated. * Starting and jumping during sleep.

**Bry.** Pain in the head, as if the *skull were being pressed asunder.* Congestion of blood to the head, with heat and burning. * Delirious talk, at night with desire to escape. Lips dry and parched, with great thirst. * Wants to keep perfectly still, as the least motion makes him worse. Sudden starting up from sleep. * Sitting up in bed causes nausea and fainting. * Constipation of dry, hard stools, as if burnt. Very irritable.

**Cimic.** Intense pressing, throbbing pain in the head, mostly in the vertex and occiput, with delirium. * Sensation as if the brain was too large for the skull, *and as if the top of the head would fly off.* Severe pain in the eyeballs. Swelling in the back part of the tongue.

**Cup. act.** If the disease has arisen from the retrocession of some acute eruption. Fretfulness or apathy. Restless or disturbed sleep. Inability to hold the head erect. Convulsive movements and distortions of the limbs. * When drinking, the fluid descends with a gurgling noise. Grinding of the teeth.

**Hell.** Usually in the last stage, when serous exudation has already taken place. * Face pale and puffed. * Soporous sleep, with screaming and starting. * Lower jaw sinking down. * Chewing motions with the mouth. * Automatic motions with one arm and one leg. Squinting, pupils dilated.

**Hyos.** Drowsiness and loss of consciousness. Indistinct speech. Delirium with wild staring look, jerking of the limbs and throbbing of the carotids. White coated tongue; *frothing at the mouth.* * Staring, distorted eyes, with double **vision**. **Starting up suddenly from sleep. * Muttering, with picking at the bed-clothes. Involuntary stools and urine.**

**Opium**. Lethargy, with stertorous breathing, eyes half closed. Stupefaction after waking. * Delirious talking, eyes wide open. Face purplish and swollen. * Acuteness of hearing. Fearfulness and great tendency to start. After grief, fright, or violent mental emotions. * Constipation, stools round, hard, black balls.

**Stram**. Great indifference. He does not notice the objects around him. Stupefaction of the senses. * Loquacious delirium, with desire to escape out of bed. * Awakens with a shrinking look, as if afraid of the first object seen. Disposed to talk continually. * Grinding of the teeth, with shuddering. Lips sore and cracked, and sordes on the teeth. *Glistening eyes and staring look.* Black fluid stools.

---

## ENTERITIS.

**Therapeutics.** Special indications.

**Acon**. In the early stage, presenting a high inflammatory fever, dry hot skin, and full frequent pulse. Mouth and tongue dry, with intense thirst. *Abdomen swollen and tender to touch.* * Cutting, burning, and tearing pains in the umbilical region, aggravated by the least pressure. * Great fear and anxiety of mind, with nervous excitability. Bright-red and hot urine.

**Ars.** Usually in the last stage. Very rapid and weak pulse. *Sudden sinking of strength*, cold, clammy sweat, and *great restlessness.* * Intense thirst, drinking often but little at a time. * Burning in the abdomen, with cutting and lancinations, *worse after eating or drinking.* Vomiting, especially after eating or drinking. Symptoms all worse after midnight.

**Bell.** Great *heat and tenderness* of the abdomen. Violent contractive, or clutching pains in the bowels.

* Pains which appear suddenly, and cease as suddenly. Congestion of blood to the head, with throbbing of the carotids. * Face flushed, eyes red and sparkling. * Great intolerance to noise and light. Starting and jumping during sleep. Sleepiness, but cannot sleep. Almost constant moaning. Partial or general spasms, with unconsciousness.

**Bry.** Inflammation, with hard swelling around the umbilicus. * Stitching or lancinating in the bowels, worse from the slightest motion. * Lies perfectly still, don't want to move. * Cannot sit up on account of nausea and faintness. *Lips parched, dry, and cracked.* Great thirst for large draughts of water. Vomiting immediately after eating or drinking. * Constipation of hard, dry stools as if burnt. Very *irritable*, everything makes him angry. Delirium, wants to get out of bed and go home.

**Canth.** Heat and burning in the abdomen and bowels, which are very *sensitive to pressure.* Cutting burning pains through the bowels. * Violent burning thirst, with aversion to all kind of drinks. * Tenesmus of the bladder, with ineffectual efforts to urinate. Stools pale-reddish mucous, like scrapings of the intestines. *Anxious restlessness.*

**Merc.** Abdomen swollen, hard, and *painful to contact.* Cutting, stabbing pains in the bowels, accompanied by chilliness and shuddering. * Green or bloody mucous stools, with violent tenesmus. * Profuse perspiration affording no relief. Pale, wretched complexion. Foul smell from the mouth; vomiting of bitter mucus. *Restless sleep.* Vomiting of bitter or bilious mucus.

---

## ERYSIPELAS.

**Therapeutics.** Special indications.

**Acon.** Chill and synochal fever, with dry hot skin and full quick pulse. Great redness, tingling, and burning in the face. Chilliness with internal heat.

* Vertigo from sitting up in bed. * Great fear and anxiety of mind, with great nervous excitability. * Cannot bear the pain, nor to be touched or uncovered.

**Apis m.** Erysipelas of the face, with œdematous swelling. * Burning, stinging pains in the affected parts. Pressing pain in the forehead and temples, worse when sitting or in a warm room. * Chilliness from the least motion, with heat of the face and hands. * Dryness of the throat without thirst. Urine dark-colored and scanty.

**Ars.** When the parts assume a *blackish hue, with a tendency to gangrene.* * Burning pains, the parts burn like fire. * Rapid prostration of strength. * Great anguish, extreme restlessness, and fear of death. * Intense thirst, drinking little and often. Worse at night, *particularly after midnight.*

**Bell.** Especially in facial erysipelas. * Smooth shining skin, not much swollen. * The redness begins in a small spot, and runs in streaks from the centre. * Congestion of blood to the head, with delirium and throbbing of the carotids. *Throbbing headache,* worse from motion. * Great intolerance of light or noise. Aggravation about 3 P. M.

**Bry.** If the disease attacks the joints. Hot, red swelling of the affected parts, with inability to move them. * Pains stitching, burning, and stinging; worse from the least motion or touch. * Patient wants to remain perfectly quiet. * Cannot sit up from nausea and faintness. *Lips parched, dry, and cracked.* Headache as if it would split open. Very irritable and impatient. *Dry, hard stools* as if burnt.

**Graph.** Unhealthy skin; the slightest injury inclines to suppurate. * Phlegmonous erysipelas of the head and face, with burning, tingling pains. * Vesicular eruptions, discharging a sticky glutinous fluid. Persons inclined to obesity.

**Hepar.** Where the disease inclines to terminate in suppuration. The eruption is very sensitive to touch. Especially after the abuse of mercury. *Empty feeling at the stomach.*

**Opium.** Cases which supervene during *pneumonia,*

typhoid or other fevers. * Profound coma, with stertorous respiration. General appearance stupid and besotted. Eyes dull and watery, pupils dilated. Face dark-red and bloated. Stools composed of hard black balls. Slow pulse.

**Puls.** *Erratic erysipelas,* where the redness disappears in one place to reappear in another. Hard, bluish-red swelling, with burning heat, and stinging, particularly when touching or moving the part. * Vertigo when rising from a sitting posture, with chilliness. Thickly coated tongue, with *very bad taste in the morning. Mild, tearful* persons, with blue eyes and blonde hair.

**Rhus.** * Vesicular erysipelas. Burning and redness of the surface, which soon swells and becomes covered with *watery vesicles.* * *Intolerable burning, itching, and tingling* in the affected parts. Swelling and redness of the face, with partial or entire closure of the eyelids. Bruised feeling in the limbs and back. Amelioration from moving the affected parts.

**Sulph.** In cases terminating in ulceration, and where it has assumed a chronic form. The parts burn and itch when near the fire, or from getting in a heat. * Frequent weak faint spells. Vesicular eruptions filled with *pus.* * Constant heat on top of the head. Early morning diarrhœa. Dry, husky, scaly skin. *Scrofulous diathesis.*

---

## GASTRITIS.

**Therapeutics.** Special indications.

**Acon.** Synochal fever, evinced by hot, dry skin, full quick pulse, and *intense thirst.* Sharp, shooting pains in the stomach, which is tender to touch. * Bitter bilious vomiting, with anguish and fear of death. Everything except water has a bitter taste. * Great fear and anxiety of mind, with great nervous excitability. Shortness of breath ; great restlessness.

**Arn.** If caused from a blow or some mechanical

injury. Painful pressure in the stomach, with pinching, spasmodic, griping pains. * Vomiting of dark coagulated blood. * Sore, bruised feeling all through the body. Belching, with taste of *putrid eggs*. Complains all the while of the bed being too hard, and keeps changing about continually.

**Ars.** Anxious expression of countenance. Great tenderness of the epigastric region to pressure. * Heat, or burning in the stomach, with sharp, shooting pains. * Vomiting of everything eaten or drank. *During the vomiting violent pain in the stomach.* * Urgent thirst for cold water, drinks often but little at a time. * Great restlessness and anxiety, with fear of death. *Rapid prostration of strength.*

**Bell.** Great tenderness of the whole abdomen, with painful pressure in the stomach. Burning and cutting pains in the stomach. * Pains which come on suddenly and cease as suddenly. Congestion of blood to the head, with throbbing headache. Delirium, with desire to escape from bed. * Great intolerance to light and noise. * Starting and jumping during sleep. Sleepiness but cannot sleep.

**Bry.** Region of the stomach exceedingly sensitive; *cannot bear the least pressure on it.* Stitching and darting pains in the pit of the stomach. *Burning in the stomach.* * Vomiting immediately after eating or drinking. * Nausea and faintness from sitting up in bed. Delirium, with desire to escape from bed and go home. Lips parched, dry, and cracked. Thirst for large draughts of cold water. * Wants to remain perfectly quiet. *Hard, dry stools, as if burnt.*

**Canth.** Violent pains in the stomach; the patient tossing about in despair. *Severe burning in the stomach,* sometimes extending down into the bowels. * Constant desire to urinate, passing but a few drops at a time. Stools like scrapings of the intestines. Burning thirst. * Vomiting, with violent retching and severe colic. Anxious restlessness.

**Ipec.** Where nausea and vomiting are the most prominent features. Diarrhœa, with *grass-green mucous stools,* and cutting colic.

**Iris v.** *Great burning distress in the epigastric region.*

Intense burning in the region of the pancreas. * Sharp cutting pains of short duration, and changing often. Distressing nausea and vomiting, with pain in the stomach. Aggravation by motion.

**Nux v.** Face red and bloated. Tongue red, clean, and tremulous. *Burning pain in the stomach*, which is very tender to touch. * Contractive, spasmodic pains in the stomach. * Vomiting of sour-smelling mucus, also of blood. Burning in the œsophagus up to the mouth. Constipation of hard, difficult stools, with frequent urging. All worse in the morning; cannot sleep after 3 A. M. Victims of drastic medicines and quack nostrums.

**Puls.** Epigastrium sensitive and painful to pressure. Aching and darting pains in the stomach. Nausea and vomiting after eating or drinking. * Suffocating and fainting spells, must have fresh, cool air. * Vertigo when rising up, with chilliness. Watery diarrhœa, especially at night. Mild, tearful disposition. Bitter taste, constant spitting of frothy mucus.

**Verat. alb.** * Hippocratic countenance. Eyes sunken and glazed. Lips bluish and dry. Great soreness in the region of the stomach. * Intense thirst for *cold drinks*. Inability to retain anything on the stomach. Extremities cold and covered with clammy sweat. *Extreme prostration*, with anguish and fear of death. *Pulse almost imperceptible. Exhausting diarrhœa.*

---

## HEADACHE.

**Therapeutics.** Special indications.

**Acon.** Violent stupefying headache, with great fulness and heaviness in the forehead. * Sensation as if the brain would press through the forehead. * Vertigo when rising from a sitting posture. Bitter bilious vomiting, with anguish and fear of death. * Gets desperate, and declares he cannot bear the pains.

**Argen. nit.** Dull, pressing pain in the forehead,

with *vertigo early in the morning.* Stupefying dulness of the head, with *great weakness of mind.* The headache is usually attended with chilliness and trembling of the body. Faintish sick feeling ending in real vomiting. Worse in the open air, and relieved by tying something tight around the head.

**Arnica.** Headache principally *over the eyes.* Stitching, darting pains in the forehead, worse by stooping. * Head and face hot, while the body is cool. * Soreness in the stomach, and belchings tasting like putrid eggs. Nausea and vomiting, worse after eating or drinking. If caused by a blow, or concussion of the brain.

**Ars.** Periodical headache. *Great weight in the head,* particularly in the forehead. *Beating pain in the forehead,* with inclination to vomit. * Violent vomiting, particularly after eating or drinking. * Extreme thirst, drinking little and often. * Restlessness, prostration, fear of death. Pains worse during rest, and better by motion.

**Bell.** Face flushed and eyes injected. Congestion of blood to the head, with throbbing of the carotids. * Violent throbbing pain, especially in the forehead, obliging one to close the eyes. * Boring headache in the right side of the head. * Vertigo, with stupefaction and vanishing of sight. *Nausea and vomiting of bile, mucus, or food.* * Cannot bear noise or bright light. Aggravation about 3 P. M.

**Bry.** Headache sets in on first waking in the morning. Beating, jerking, or stitching pains, especially on one side. * The head aches as if it would split open, aggravated by stooping or motion. * Wants to keep perfectly still. Sour or bitter vomiting. Thickly coated tongue; lips parched, dry, and cracked. * Constipation of hard dry stools as if burnt. Patient very irritable.

**Cactus.** Headache from irregular habits or dissipation. Pulsating pain, with a sensation of weight in the right side of the head. Pain commencing in the morning and growing worse as the day advances. Must lie perfectly quiet, as any motion, noise, or light increases the suffering.

**Calc. c.** Chronic headache. Dull, stupefying, oppressive pain in the forehead, with cloudiness of intellect. Throbbing headache in the morning, continuing the whole day. * Feeling of coldness in the head. * Feet cold as if they had on damp stockings. * Much dandruff on the scalp. Vertigo on going up stairs. Menses *too soon, too profuse,* and *lasting too long.*

**Cham.** If caused from catarrh, or by drinking coffee. Rending or drawing pain in one side of the head extending to the jaw. Acute shooting or throbbing pains in the forehead. * One cheek red and the other pale. * Bitter bilious vomiting. *Over-sensitive to pain;* gets almost furious. * Very impatient, can hardly answer one civilly. Dysmenorrhœa, with labor-like pains.

**China.** Headache from suppressed coryza. Pressure in the forehead as if it would burst. Soreness of the brain as if bruised, worse from mental exertion. * Intense throbbing headache after excessive depletion. * Ringing in the ears, and weak fainting spells. Worse every other day.

**Cocc.** Sick-headache from riding in a carriage, on a boat, &c. Tearing, throbbing headache, especially in the evening. * Violent headache, which compels the patient to sit up, aggravated by *talking, laughing, noise, or a bright light.* * Vertigo, with nausea and vomiting from the motion of a carriage. Constipation of hard difficult stools. Dysmenorrhœa followed by hemorrhoids.

**Coffea.** Patient very sensitive and excitable. * Headache as if a nail were driven into the brain, worse in the open air. Pain in the head as if it would fly to pieces, worse from noise or light. *Head feels too small.* * Extreme wakefulness. Burning, sour eructations.

**Glonoin.** Congestive nervous headache, with no gastric or bilious symptoms. * Violent *throbbing, pulsating headache,* with fulness and upward pressure in the head. * Undulating sensation in the head, worse from turning round. *Sick, faint-like feeling at the stomach, with nausea.* Head feels too large. Palpitation of the heart. *Sun-stroke.*

**Igna.** Boring, sticking pain in the forehead, relieved by lying down. * Pain as if a nail were driven out through the side of the head, relieved by lying on it. Headache as if something hard pressed upon the surface of the brain. * Patient full of suppressed grief, with an empty feeling at the pit of the stomach. Constipation, with prolapsus ani.

**Ipecac.** * If nausea and vomiting is the most prominent feature. Headache as if the brain and skull were bruised even to the root of the tongue. * Stooping causes vomiting. Diarrhœa with grass-green stools.

**Lach.** Headache with nausea and drowsiness. Throbbing or beating pains in the temples. Pressing headache early in the morning, worse from stooping. * Cannot bear anything tight about the waist. Vertigo with paleness of the face. *Pain in the left ovarian region.* * Larynx and throat very sensitive to touch. Despondent mood. *Aggravation after sleeping.*

**Nux v.** Headache with sour, bitter vomiting. Pressing, *boring* pain, with sensation as if the skull would split. * Stupefying headache, especially in the morning, aggravated by mental exertion. * Habitual constipation of large difficult stools, with frequent urging. Persons of *sedentary* or *intemperate* habits, or those *troubled with piles.*

**Phos. ac.** Dreadful pain on top of the head, as though the brain were crushed, after long continued grief. * Too early and long continued menstruation, with pain in the liver. * Sensation as if the stomach were being balanced up and down. Painless diarrhœa; whitish stools.

**Puls.** Headache consequent upon eating rich, greasy food. *Tearing, drawing,* or *stitching pains,* worse towards evening. * Vertigo, especially when stooping or looking up. * Craves cool fresh air, and feels worse in a close warm room. *Nausea* and vomiting with repugnance to food. * Menses too late, scanty, or suppressed. Chilliness even in a warm room. Very bad taste in the morning. Mild, tearful disposition.

**Sang. can.** Sick-headache. * Pains in the back part of the head, running in rays from the neck upwards. Severe pains in the head, especially over the right eye, with *nausea and vomiting.* * Has to keep in a dark room and lie perfectly still.

**Sepia.** *Beating, stitching,* or jerking pains, mostly in the forehead or temples. Also, violent pain as if the head would burst, extorting cries. * Nausea and vomiting, with a feeling of emptiness in the stomach. * Dirty yellow appearance of the face, especially across the nose. Constipation, with hard, knotty stool. Very *fetid urine* depositing a clay-colored sediment. *Leucorrhœa* between the menses.

**Silicea.** Beating or throbbing pains, mostly in the forehead, with heat and congestion to the head. Tearing pains mostly on one side with stitches through the eyes. The pains are worse from mental exertion, stooping, talking, or cold air; better in a warm room. * Constipation, the stools recede after having been partially expelled.

**Spig.** Periodical headache. Pains *boring,* pressing, increased by motion, noise, and especially by *stooping.* * Nervous headache when one or both eyes are involved. * Severe pressing and sticking pains in the eyes, worse during motion. Palpitation of the heart.

**Sulph.** Pains mostly in the forehead and temples, of a pressing, throbbing, or tearing character. * Constant heat on top of the head, and coldness of the feet. * Early morning diarrhœa, driving the patient out of bed in a hurry. * Frequent weak, faint spells through the day. *Suppressed eruptions. Hemorrhoids.* * Lean persons who walk stooping.

**Verat. alb.** Nervous headache. Violent pains, that almost deprive the patient of reason. * Becomes very weak and faint, with cold perspiration all over. * Coldness on top of the head. * Vomiting with exhausting diarrhœa, and cold sweat. Nervous headache at each menstrual period. *Great thirst for cold drinks.*

## HÆMOPTYSIS.

**Therapeutics.** Special indications.

**Acon.** The attack is preceded by fulness or congestion of the chest, and burning pain. Palpitation of the heart, anguish and restlessness. * Great fear and anxiety of mind, with great nervous excitability.

**Arn.** If caused by a fall or blow on the breast or back. * Expectoration of dark and coagulated blood. Tickling under the sternum, and a sore pain as if bruised in the chest when coughing. * The bed on which he lies feels too hard.

**Bell.** * Congestion to the head and chest. Constant tickling in the larynx, with cough and expectoration of bloody mucus. Stitch-like pains in the chest, worse by motion. * Vertigo when stooping or rising from a stooping posture. Takes cold from every draught of air.

**China.** After great loss of blood or animal fluids. * Singing in the ears and fainting spells. Periodical attacks, worse every other day. *Debilitating morning* and *night sweats.*

**Dulc.** Constant titillation in the larynx, with desire to cough. Expectoration of bright-red blood. Hemorrhage caused by a cold or a loose cough which existed some time. * Gets worse at every cold change in the weather. * On waking in the morning, feels giddy and dizzy, with a sense of trembling and weakness.

**Ferr.** Hemorrhage with flying pains in the chest, better when walking slowly about. * Hæmoptysis with pain between the shoulders. Palpitation of the heart and difficult breathing. * The least emotion or exertion produces a red flushed face. Slender persons with sallow complexion.

**Hem. v.** Profuse hemorrhage; blood venous, coming into the mouth without any effort, like a warm current from out the chest. Mind calm. Sometimes taste of sulphur in the mouth. Frequent paroxysms of pain in the left ovary, passing down to the uterus.

**Hyos.** The hemorrhage is preceded by a dry

cough, especially at night, obliging the patient to sit up. * Frequent and sudden starting from sleep, with red face, and wild staring look. *Things seem too large;* frequent looking at the hands because they seem too large.

**Puls.** In obstinate cases, the discharge is black and coagulated. Loose cough. * Very nervous during the night. * Chilliness even in a warm room. Weakness and pain in the lower part of the chest. Sickish, empty feeling in the stomach. * Craves fresh cool air, worse in a warm room. Scanty or suppressed menses. Persons of a mild, tearful disposition.

**Rhus tox.** Dry cough, which seems as if it would tear something out of the chest. Discharge of light-red blood. * Tickling under the sternum, that excites the cough. After straining, lifting, or stretching the arms high up to reach things.

---

## HEMORRHOIDS.

**Therapeutics.** Special indications.

**Acon.** Bleeding piles. Stinging and pressure in the anus. General dryness of the skin. * Constant restlessness, inability to keep still. Persons of a full plethoric habit.

**Æsculus.** Large protruding tumors, with slight hemorrhage. * *Itching, burning pains,* with a sense of fulness and dryness of the anus. * Severe aching pains in the lumbar and sacral region, with stiffness of the back, aggravated by walking. *Constant backache, affecting the sacrum and hips.*

**Aloes.** Protruding piles, bleeding often and profusely. * Great heat and tenderness of the tumors, relieved by cold water. Violent tenesmus, with bloody or jelly-like mucous stools. * Fistula in ano. Dull, heavy headache, with dull pains in the liver. A feeling of faintness during and after stool.

**Apis.** Hemorrhoids, with stinging, burning, and smarting pains, relieved by cold water. * Constipation, with a sensation in the abdomen as if something tight would break, if too much effort was used to void the stool. * Enlargement of the right ovary, with pain in left pectoral region, with cough.

**Ars.** Blind piles, which *burn like fire*, particularly at night, hindering sleep. During the day, stinging pains, particularly when walking. * Great anguish, restlessness, and fear of death. Much thirst, drinks little and often. All worse at night, particularly *after midnight.*

**Bell.** Bleeding piles, with great tenderness and pain from the slightest touch. * Feeling in the back as if it would break, hindering motion. * Pains which appear suddenly and cease just as suddenly. Congestion of the head with throbbing in the temples. * Sleepy but cannot sleep. Feverish restlessness.

**Calc. c.** Varices swollen and protruded, emitting considerable blood. Burning, pricking in the rectum, so that the patient cannot remain still. Drawing, cutting pains in the rectum, with a feeling of painfulness, particularly after stool. * Menstruation too frequent and too profuse. * Cold damp feet. Vertigo on going up stairs.

**Carb. v.** Swollen, protruding varices, discharging pure blood. * Acrid corroding humor oozing from the rectum emitting a *fetid smell.* Tickling, itching, and burning of the varices. Stools of *foul bloody mucus.* * Eructations of sour rancid food, with *much flatulence* from the bowels.

**Cascarilla.** Frequent and profuse bleeding from the rectum during and after stool. Constipation of hard, brown, lumpy stools, sometimes covered with slime.

**Caust.** Large and painful varices, hindering stool. * Stinging and burning of the tumors when touched, intolerable when walking. Weak scrofulous persons, with yellow complexion. Pressure and fulness in the abdomen as if it would burst, worse after eating.

**Collinsonia.** Blind or bleeding piles, with a sensation as if *gravel or sand had lodged in the rectum.* Obstinate and habitual constipation; stools lumpy and light-colored, with dull pain in the anus. Dysmenorrhœa. Aggravation in the evening and better in the morning.

**Graph.** Hemorrhoids with prolapsus recti. Painful burning cracks between the varices. Burning, itching, and sticking in the rectum. * Prolapsus recti, without straining, as if the sphincter were paralyzed. * Chronic constipation of hard, difficult, *knotty stools.* * Unhealthy skin, and eruptions that excrete a sticky fluid.

**Hemam.** *Profusely bleeding hemorrhoids,* with burning soreness, and at times rawness of the anus. The back feels as if it would break off. * Passive hemorrhage from the nose, stomach, or bowels.

**Ignatia.** Hemorrhoids, with violent shooting pains high up in the rectum. * The tumors prolapse with every stool and have to be replaced. Soreness of the parts as if excoriated. * Bleeding and pain worse when the stool is loose. Drawing pain around the pelvis. * Full of suppressed grief, with an empty feeling at the pit of the stomach.

**Kali c.** Large, painful varices, with considerable protrusion *during micturition.* Large difficult stools, as if from inactivity. of the rectum. * The tumors swell and bleed during stool, with pricking and burning. * Constipation, with distress one or two hours before stool, with colicky stitching pains.

**Mur. ac.** Large protruding piles, with burning and sore pain. * The tumors are bluish, are *extremely sensitive and painful.* * Violent itching of the parts not relieved by scratching. Discharge of blood with the stool. Prolapsus ani during micturition.

**Nitric ac.** Bleeding piles, protruding after every stool. * Sharp cutting pain in the rectum, lasting for hours after an evacuation, and is worse after a loose stool. * Old hemorrhoidal tumors, secreting much slime, and bleeding profusely after stool. *Fissures of the anus.*

**Nux v.** Blind or bleeding piles. Burning, pricking pains in the tumors. Discharge of light-colored blood after stool. Horrid tearing, pressing pains in the small of the back and lower bowels. * Frequent ınd ineffectual urging to stool. * Habitual constipa-ion, with frequent urging to stool. Is very irritable, ınd wishes to be alone. Persons of sedentary or in-emperate habits, and the victims of drugs, nos-rums, &c.

**Puls.** Mostly *blind* piles, with painful pressure on he tumors. Stinging, itching in the rectum, and *soreness of the anus.* * Obstinate constipation, with nauseous bad taste in the morning. * Inclination to be chilly even in a warm room. * Vertigo on rising from a sitting posture. Symptoms all *worse towards evening.* Mild, tearful disposition.

**Rhus t.** Sore blind piles, protruding after every stool. Drawing in the back from above downwards; ension and pressing in the rectum. * Pain in the small of the back as if bruised, relieved by motion. Worse from getting wet, or by lifting heavy loads. Rheumatic diathesis.

**Sepia.** Mostly *bleeding* piles, with protrusion of he tumors and rectum during stool. Continual strain-ng pain in the rectum, with heat, burning, and swell-ng of the anus. Difficulty in urinating, especially in he morning. * Sense of weight or of a ball in the anus, not relieved by stool.

**Sulph.** *Blind or bleeding* piles. Constant urging o stool, which continues after a thin bloody evacua-ion. * Stinging, burning, and soreness in and about he anus. Prolapsus recti, especially during a hard stool. Violent stitching pains in the back. Burning pains in the urethra during micturition. * Weak, faint spells, especially when standing or walking. * Constant heat on top of the head. Aggravation in he morning.

---

## HEPATITIS.

**Therapeutics.** Special indications.

**Acon.** Violent inflammatory fever, with stitches n the region of the liver. * Intolerable pains driving one to despair. * Great restlessness, anxiety, and fear of death. Vertigo on sitting up in bed. Headache as if everything would press out of the forehead. Bitter bilious vomiting. * Retention of urine, with stitches in the kidneys. *Great nervous excitability.*

**Ars.** Region of the liver tender and swollen, with violent burning pains. Vomiting of *brownish* or *blackish* substances. Diarrhœa of blackish stools, worse after eating or drinking. * Violent thirst, drinking little and often. Great anguish, restlessness, and fear of death. *Rapid prostration* of strength.

**Bell.** Acute pain in the region of the liver, extending to the chest and shoulder. Tension in the region of the stomach. Labored and anxious breathing. * Tenderness of the whole abdomen, aggravated by the least jar, even of the bed on which he lies. * Congestion of the head, with throbbing pains in the temples. Almost constant moaning; the patient seems drowsy, with *starting and jumping during sleep.* * Delirium, with desire to escape. Cannot bear noise or bright light.

**Bry.** Burning or stitching pains in the hypochondria. Pain in the right shoulder and arm. Yellow-coated tongue, with bitter, bilious vomiting. * Lips cracked, parched, and dry. Headache as if it would split open. * Sitting up in bed causes nausea and faintness. Region of the stomach very sensitive to touch or pressure. * Exceedingly irritable, everything makes him angry. * Constipation of hard, dry stools, as if burnt. * Wants to keep perfectly quiet.

**Chelido.** Acute or dull pain, and tenderness of the region of the liver. * Constant pain under the lower inner angle of the right shoulder-blade. Sallow, jaundiced complexion. Pressive pain in the back part of the head, towards the left ear. * Stools like sheep's dung, or soft and bright yellow. Urine scanty, deep yellow, and sour.

**Lep. vir.** Aching pains in the liver. Yellow-coated tongue. Black, profuse, papescent, tar-like, very fetid stools, generally in the afternoon or evening. Dark-brown urine. Constant distress in the lower part of the epigastrium.

**Merc.** Pressive pain and stitches in the liver. Inability to lie on the right side. * Inflammation, with great tenderness of the liver to contact, and jaundice-like appearance of the skin. * When coughing or sneezing, a stitch runs directly through the chest to the back. * Much perspiration affording no relief. *Green, bilious,* or frothy stools, with *frequent urging* and *tenesmus.* Bilious vomiting.

**Nux v.** Stitching or throbbing pains in the liver, with great tenderness to contact. * Sour or bitter taste in the mouth, with bilious vomiting. Shortness of breath, and sense of pressure under the ribs. * Headache as if it would split open. Habitual constipation of large difficult stools. * Cannot sleep after 3 A. M. Symptoms all worse in the morning. Persons of sedentary or intemperate habits.

**Podo. pel.** Fulness and pain in the region of the liver. Nausea and bilious vomiting. * The patient is constantly rubbing and shaking the hypochondriac region. Bitter taste and risings in the mouth. * Painless morning diarrhœa.

**Puls.** Yellow-coated tongue, and bitter taste in the mouth. Frequent attacks of anguish, especially at night. Nausea and desire to vomit. * Green, slimy diarrhœa, usually at night. * Chilliness, even in a warm room, with vertigo when rising from a sitting posture. Persons of a *mild, tearful* disposition. Frequent urging to urinate, with cutting pain. Symptoms all worse towards evening.

**Silicea.** Hardness and distention of the region of the liver. Throbbing ulcerative pain, increased by contact and motion. * Formation of abscess. * Constipation, the stool recedes after having been partially expelled. * Lymphatic swellings, with inclination to suppurate.

**Sulph.** Mostly chronic hepatitis. Swelling and hardness of the liver. Beating, stitching pains and pressure in the liver. Sour or bitter taste. * Frequent weak, faint spells, with flashes of heat. * Constant heat on top of the head. Constipation, or *early morning diarrhœa.* * Drowsy during the day, and wakeful the whole night.

## HYDROCEPHALUS.

**Therapeutics.** Special indications.

**Acon.** In the early stage, when the febrile excitement runs high. * Intolerance to light and noise. * Great fear and anxiety, with nervous excitability. * The child is sleepless, restless, cries much, bites its fist, and has a green watery diarrhœa.

**Apis m.** High fever with delirium. Sleep interrupted by sudden shrill cries. * Boring the head deep into the pillow. * Squinting, and grinding the teeth. * Twitching on one side of the body, while the other is paralyzed. Profuse perspiration on the head. Frequent and scanty emissions of urine.

**Apo. can.** Sutures open. Forehead projecting. Sight of one eye totally lost, and the other slightly sensible. Stupor. Constant involuntary motion of one leg and arm. Urine suppressed. Compare with *Hellebore.*

**Artemisia.** Convulsions of the right side, and paralysis of the left. Body cold all over. Sopor, yet drinking and swallowing water eagerly. Face pale, with an oldish look. Involuntary stools, which are greenish and thin.

**Bell.** Face flushed and eyes injected. Boring with the head in the pillow, rolling the eyes and squinting. * Throbbing of the carotids. * Sudden starting and jumping during sleep. Delirium, with desire to get out of bed. Involuntary emissions of urine. *Great intolerance of light or noise.*

**Bry.** Manifest *signs of effusion.* Dark flushed face, dry and parched lips. Tongue coated with a dark-yellowish fur. * Frequent motion of the jaws, as if chewing something. * Cannot sit up on account of nausea and faintness. * Constipation of hard, dry stools, as if burnt. Scanty, hot, red urine. Exceedingly irritable.

**Calc. c.** Persons of a scrofulous diathesis. * Large head, with open fontanelles. * Profuse perspiration on the head when sleeping. * Emaciation with a good appetite. Painful and difficult urination, the urine having a strong fetid odor.

**Hell.** After exudation has taken place. * Automatic motions of one arm and one leg. * Soporous sleep, with screaming and starting. * Lower jaw sinking down. Chewing motion with the mouth. Squinting, pupils dilated. Forehead drawn in folds, and covered with cold perspiration. Vomiting of green or blackish substances.

**Opium.** * Extreme drowsiness, and coma, with stertorous breathing. The face is purplish and swollen. * Screaming before or during the spasm. Depression of the lower jaw. Dilated or contracted pupils, and general symptoms of paralysis of the brain.

**Stram.** Convulsive motions of the head. Sensation of lightness in the head, causing the patient to frequently raise it up. * Awakens with a shrinking look as if afraid of the first object seen. * Loquacious delirium, with a desire to escape. No thirst, although the mouth is very dry. * Light of brilliant objects, and contact renew the spasms. Stools black fluid.

**Sulph.** Heaviness of the head, sinking involuntary backwards. Sweat on the head, with a kind of musk-like smell. Frequent change of color in the face. Sour smell from the mouth. * Drowsiness in the daytime and wakefulness at night. Scrofulous diathesis; dry, husky, scaly skin. * After suppressed or dried-up eruptions on the head, behind the ears, or elsewhere.

**Zinc.** *Impending paralysis* of the brain. Frequent jerking of the whole body, and crying out during sleep. When awakened, expresses fear, and rolls his head from side to side. * Constant trembling of the hands, with coldness of the extremities. Gagging and vomiting, with a voracious appetite.

---

## INTERMITTENT FEVER.

**Therapeutics.** Special indications.

**Acon.** In recent cases of young persons of full habit. Violent chill, and heat especially about the head and face. *Great fear and anxiety of mind, with great nervous excitability. Palpitation of the heart, and pleuritic stitches in the chest.

**Ant. c.** Much gastric disturbance. White coated tongue. *Great sadness and a woful mood. *Chilliness predominates.* Great desire to sleep; want of thirst.

**Apis m.** Chill about 4 P. M., worse in a warm room or near a stove. Renewed chilliness from the slightest motion, with heat of the face and hands. Sweat alternating with dryness of the skin. During the apyrexia, pain under the short ribs, worse on the left side. *Sensation in the abdomen as if something tight would break, if much effort were made to void a stool.

**Arnica.** Chill in the evening. Thirst before and during the chill. During the fever, constant desire to change one's position. *Sore, bruised feeling all through the body, as if he had been beaten. *The bed or couch on which he lies feels *too hard.* Eructations smelling like bad eggs.

**Ars.** Paroxysms imperfectly developed. Before the chill, vertigo, headache, yawning, stretching, and general discomfort. The chill is frequently intermingled with heat and fever; or there is internal chilliness and external heat at the same time. *During the fever, great anguish, extreme restlessness, and fear of death. After the paroxysm, *great prostration.* *Urgent thirst, drinking often but little at a time.

**Bell.** *Slight chill*, with *much fever*, or vice versa. Some parts are cold, while others are warm. Violent throbbing headache, with stupefaction. *Heat and red face, with throbbing of the carotids. Choking sensation in the throat, with dryness of the mouth.

**Bry.** The chill predominates. Great thirst during all the stages. *Violent, dry, racking cough, with stitching pains in the side of the chest. Stitching pain in the region of the liver and abdomen. *Constipation of hard, dry stools, as if burnt. Exceedingly irritable; everything makes him angry.

**Cactus.** Chill at 11 A. M., or 11 P. M. First chill, then burning heat, with headache, coma, stupefacion, insensibility. Thirst, shortness of breath, inability to remain lying. Profuse sweat, attended with unquenchable thirst.

**Calc. c.** Persons of a scrofulous diathesis. Thirst during the chill. Chills alternating with heat, or external coldness and internal heat. Hardness of hearing. * Feet feel as if they had on cold, damp stockings. Patient very weakly in general; vertigo and shortness of breath on going up stairs. Diarrhœa, stools whitish, undigested.

**Cap. an.** Chill with thirst, followed by heat without thirst. * The chill commences in the back and from thence extends over the entire body. Drowsiness during the fever accompanied by perspiration. Much pain in the back and limbs.

**Carb. v.** Paroxysms irregular, sometimes commencing with sweat followed by chill. The attack is preceded or attended by toothache and pain in the limbs. * Thirst only during the chilly stage. Vertigo, redness of the face and sick stomach during the hot stage. * When eating or drinking, sensation as if the stomach or abdomen would burst.

**Cedron.** Chills and shiverings very severe, with cramps, and tearing pains in the upper and lower extremities. Dry heat, followed by profuse perspiration. * Numb, dead feeling in the legs; they feel enlarged. * The entire body feels numb.

**Cham.** Chill generally light. Heat and sweat predominate. Much thirst in the hot stage. * Face red, or one cheek red and the other pale. * Very impatient, can hardly answer one civilly. Hot perspiration about the head and face. * Pain in the abdomen, with frequent emissions of large quantities of pale urine.

**China.** The paroxysm is preceded by nausea, headache, hunger, anguish, and palpitation of the heart. * Thirst before the chill. and during the sweating stage. Chills alternating with heat, skin cold and blue. Ringing in the ears, with dizziness and a feeling as if the head was enlarged. * Pain in the region of the liver and spleen, when bending or coughing. Sallow complexion. Miasmatic districts.

**Cimex.** *Before* the *chill* thirst and heaviness in the legs. *Chill* commences with clenching of the hands and violent raging. *During the chill,* pains in all the joints. Sensation as if the tendons were too short. *During the heat,* gagging. Thirst, but drinking causes violent headache. *The sweat* is mostly on the head and chest, accompanied by hunger.

**Cina.** Vomiting and great hunger before, during, or after the paroxysm. Thirst only during the chill or heat. Pale face throughout the paroxysm. Frequent tickling in the nose. Restless at night. * Dilatation of the pupils; perfectly clean tongue.

**Eupato. per.** Thirst several hours before the chill, continuing during the chill and heat. Stiffness of the fingers during the chill. The paroxysm usually occurs about 7 or 9 A. M. * During the chill severe aching in the back and limbs as if the bones were broken. Sweat not very prominent. * Vomiting of whatever is eaten or drank.

**Eupato. pur.** * Chill commencing in the back, and then spreading over the body. * Violent shaking, with comparatively little coldness. Thirst during the chill and heat. Violent pain in the bones during the chill and heat. Head feels light, and as if it was falling to the left side.

**Ferr.** Chill with thirst, headache, and swelling of the cutaneous veins. Œdema of the face, especially around the eyes. Vomiting of everything eaten without being digested. * The least emotion or exertion produces a red flushed face. *Great loss of muscular power.* In protracted and badly treated cases by quinine.

**Gels.** Chill mostly in the evening, commencing in the extremities. The heat is attended with nervous restlessness and mental anxiety. Vertigo, with a sense of intoxication as if he would fall down. Sensitive to light or noise.

**Hepar.** Chill generally in the evening, preceded by bitter taste in the mouth. Chill followed by heat with sweat, especially on the chest and forehead, with slight thirst. * Itching, stinging nettle-rash before and during the chill. *Fever blisters around* the *mouth.* Previous abuse of mercury.

**Ignatia.** Thirst *only* during the chill. External heat with partial internal shuddering. * *The chill is relieved by external* heat. Very little perspiration, or only in the face. Headache and pain in the pit of the stomach.

**Ipecac.** Much chilliness with little heat, or much heat and little chilliness. Paroxysm sets in with yawning, stretching, and a collection of saliva in the mouth. Chill increases by external heat. No thirst in the cold stage, but a great deal in the hot. * *Nausea and vomiting* predominate. The *apyrexia* is marked by more or less gastric disturbance.

**Lach.** Paroxysm usually in the afternoon. The chill predominates. * Much chattering of the teeth, with violent headache and soreness in the chest. * Patient desires to be held on account of the violence of the chill hurting the head and chest. After previous abuse of quinine. * Can bear nothing to touch the throat or neck.

**Lyc.** * The paroxysm comes on about 4 P. M., and terminates about 8 P. M. * Constant sense of fulness in the stomach and abdomen as though they would burst. Obstinate constipation. * Red sediment like sand in the urine. Great fear of being left alone.

**Natr. m.** * Chill commencing at 10 A. M., with great thirst, drinking often and much at a time. During the heat violent headache. * Dry tongue, and ulcerated corners of the mouth.

**Nux v.** Paroxysm usually at night or early in the morning. * Long-lasting, hard chill, with bluish cold face and blue finger-nails. * Great heat, notwithstanding the patient wants to be covered all the while. Both chill and heat are accompanied with gastric and bilious symptoms. *During the chill*, pain in the sacrum. *During the fever*, headache, vertigo, red face, pain in the chest and vomiting.

**Opi.** Drowsiness or heavy sleep, with loud snoring during the cold and hot stages. * Stertorous respiration, with the mouth wide open. Congestion of blood to the head, with red and puffy appearance of the face. Aged persons and children.

**Puls.** The attack mostly occurs in the afternoon or evening. *Chill* and *heat* simultaneous. *No thirst* during the entire paroxysm, or only in the hot stage. Bitter or sour vomiting of mucus or bile. * Thickly coated tongue, and *bad taste in the morning.* Slight disorder of the stomach induces a relapse. * Much gastric disturbance. Persons of a mild, tearful disposition.

**Rhus t.** Paroxysm usually in the after part of the day. Chill preceded by stretching of the limbs and yawning. Coldness of some parts of the body, and heat in others. Perspiration after midnight or towards morning. During the hot stage, nettle - rash breaks out. * Restlessness, constantly changing position. * Dry, teasing cough, coming on before, and continuing during the chill.

**Sabad.** Chill predominates, with thirst between the chill and heat. * The paroxysm recurs at the same hour on each or alternate days. * Dry, hacking cough during the chill. During the apyrexia, constant chilliness.

**Samb.** * Profuse debilitating perspiration, even in the apyrexia. Cold creeps over the whole body, with fine stitching formication. Icy-cold hands and feet. Burning heat in the face, with moderately warm body and cold feet.

**Sepia.** General cold feeling, with pressure over the temples and eyes. * Great coldness of the hands, with sensation as if the *fingers were dead.* During the heat, vertigo, even to insensibility. Sweating over the whole body, with anxiety, and dryness of the throat. * Perfect absence of thirst.

**Sulph.** Attacks mostly in the evening or at night, preceded by thirst and lassitude. Chilliness in the back, chest, and arms, with coldness of the hands, feet, and nose. During the heat, thirst with burning in the hands and feet, and a bruised, tired feeling in the limbs. * Burning heat on top of the head. * Frequent weak, faint spells through the day. * Early morning diarrhœa.

**Verat. alb.** Severe chill, with feeling of internal heat, or both together. Great thirst, especially during the chill, and sweating. Profuse *sweat, often cold* and long continued. * Great exhaustion and sinking of strength. Vomiting and diarrhœa. Intermittents during the prevalence of cholera.

---

## JAUNDICE.

**Therapeutics.** Special indications.

**Acon.** Synochal fever, with acute stitches in the region of the liver. Yellowish color of the skin. Scanty red urine. *Great fear and anxiety of mind, with nervous excitability.

**Ars.** Yellowness of the skin and sclerotica. Undigested, light-colored, offensive stools. * Great anguish, restlessness, and fear of death. * Urgent thirst, drinks often but little at a time. Irritable mood, alternating with lowness of spirits.

**Berberis.** Icterus, with pale, tough alvine, or profuse acrid, watery diarrhœa. * Urine dark-yellow, with copious sediment. Morbid hunger, or loathing of food. Pressure in the region of the liver. Bloatedness of the abdomen.

**Bry.** Stitching pains in the liver when pressed upon. Pain in the right shoulder and arm. Pain in the limbs, worse by motion. Yellow-coated tongue, with bitter bilious vomiting. * Lips parched, dry, and cracked. Nausea and faintness on sitting up. *Constipation, stools dry and hard as if burnt.

**Calc. c.** Patient of a scrofulous habit. * Large head and open fontanelles. Stitches in the liver during or after stooping. Enlargement of the liver. Cannot bear tight clothing around the hypochondria. * Clay-like stools, scant and knotty. Fetid, dark-brown urine, white sediment. * Cold, damp feet. Swollen abdomen; emaciation and good appetite.

**Cham.** Mostly new-born children, or after chagrin. Yellowness of the face and whites of the eyes. * Green, watery, corroding stools, with colic. Bitter taste with bilious vomiting. * Very impatient, can hardly answer one civilly. * Children are very cross and fretful, and want to be carried all the time.

**China.** Persons who have been weakened by loss of animal fluids. *Yellow color of the skin.* Dulness and muddled condition of the head. Oppressive, tearing headache. Liver swollen, hard and tender. * Bitter taste in the back part of the throat, everything tastes bitter. * Abdomen feels full and tight as if stuffed. Yellow, watery, undigested stools, without pain. *Aggravation every other day.*

**Dig.** Frequent and empty retching, with a clean tongue. Soreness and bloatedness of the pit of the stomach. * Stools almost white. Frequent and *painful* emissions of *scanty, brown urine. Irregular or intermittent pulse.*

**Iodine.** * Yellow, almost dark-brown color of the face. Thickly coated tongue. White diarrhœic stools alternating with constipation. *Dark, yellowish-green, corroding urine.* Nausea and thirst. After mercurial poisoning.

**Mag. m.** Induration of the liver, with pressive pain extending to the back and stomach. Face dirty, dark-yellow. Tongue dirty yellowish. Bowels distended and hard, with pressure and heaviness. Stools hard and of a grayish color. Palpitation of the heart. Œdema of the feet and legs. Weak and emaciated.

**Merc.** Painfulness of the region of the liver, *skin very yellow.* * Grayish-white fæces, with tenesmus during and after stool. Thickly coated flabby tongue. * Bad smell from the mouth. Nausea and vomiting. Loathing of food. Urine scanty and red, with a strong smell.

**Nux v.** Sour or putrid taste in the mouth, with aversion to food. Contractive pain in the region of the liver. Nausea and bilious vomiting. * Constipation, with unsuccessful urging to stool. * Cannot sleep after 3 A. M. * Very irritable and wishes to be alone. Aggravation in the morning. Persons of sedentary or intemperate habits.

**Puls.** Yellow coating on the tongue, with bitter taste in the mouth. Nausea and desire to vomit. Frequent attacks of anguish, especially at night. * Chilliness, with vertigo on rising from a sitting posture. * Green, slimy diarrhœa, especially at night. *Thirstlessness.* Mild, tearful disposition. Aggravation towards evening.

**Sulph.** Beating, stitching pains in the region of the liver. Sour or bitter taste in the mouth. Abdomen bloated. * Weak, faint spells, and flashes of heat. * Constant heat on top of the head. Itching of the skin at night. * Drowsy during the day and wakeful at night. Constipation, or *morning diarrhœa.* Scrofulous diathesis.

---

## LABOR.

Strictly speaking, labor is a natural physiological process; frequently, however, cases occur in which it is protracted much beyond the usual period, or is attended with a great amount of suffering; in such cases, recourse to the following remedies will greatly relieve or remove the difficulty.

**Therapeutics.** Special indications.

**Cham.** Over-excitement, and excessive sensibility to pain. Anguish and discouragement, with tossing about. * Pains spasmodic and very distressing. * She is very impatient, can hardly answer a civil question.

**Coff.** Pains excessively violent, with great mental and general nervous excitement. * She weeps and laments fearfully. * Great sensitiveness of the genital organs, cannot bear them to be touched. *Great wakefulness at night.*

**Ign.** Hysterical fitful women, and who are full of grief. * Weak, empty feeling in the stomach, not relieved by eating. Uterine cramps, with cutting stitches. Convulsive jerking in single parts or limbs. * Patient seems full of grief, with frequent sighing.

**Nux v.** Pains irregular, and the labor does not seem to advance. Drawing in the back and thighs with pressure downwards. * Every pain produces a desire to go to stool or to urinate. Habitual constipation, with frequent urging to stool. Irritable temper.

**Opium.** Persons of full habit, and when the pains suddenly cease. Determination of blood to the head, with bloated, red face. * Drowsiness and delirious talking. Bed feels so hot she cannot lie upon it.

**Puls.** The pains seem too weak and too far apart, they grow weaker as if from inactivity of the womb. * Pains which excite palpitation of the heart, or suffocating, fainting spells. * Patient craves cool, fresh air, worse in a warm room. Mild, tearful women, with blue eyes and light hair.

**Secale.** * The pain is much prolonged, as if pressing and forcing the uterus. * Constant sensation of bearing down in the abdomen; or the pains are too weak or suppressed. * Thin, scrawny women, subject to passive hemorrhages. Desire to be uncovered; worse in a warm room.

**Cimicifu.** This remedy, given once daily for ten or twelve days *previous* to the expected confinement, is said to greatly facilitate labor and shorten its duration.

---

## LEUCORRHŒA.

**Therapeutics.** Special indications.

**Asculus.** * Constant backache affecting the sacrum and hips. * Great fatigue from walking ever so little, on account of the weakness in the back. Large protruding hemorrhoids, and constipation.

**Alumina.** Leucorrhœa just before or after the menses. * Profuse, purulent, yellowish, corroding discharge, relieved by cold applications. Severe burning pain in the small of the back. Great inactivity of the rectum, with much straining at stool.

**Amb. gris.** Discharge of bluish-white mucus. * Leucorrhœa only at night. * Stitches in the vagina preceding the discharge. Nervous hysterical subjects. During micturition, burning, smarting, itching in the vulva.

**Amm. m.** Leucorrhœa, with distention of the abdomen. * Discharge like the white of egg, preceded by a pinching pain around the navel. * Brown, slimy leucorrhœa after urinating. Intolerable pain in the small of the back at night. Menses premature, profuse, and composed of black clots.

**Ars.** Acrid, corroding leucorrhœa. * Discharge thick, yellow, dropping out while standing, or when emitting flatus. Great anguish and restlessness at night. Feeble, weakly women.

**Bovista.** Especially *after* the catamenia. * Discharge like the white of egg, coming away while walking. Also, yellowish, green, corrosive leucorrhœa. Menses too often and too profuse, with painful bearing down towards the genitals.

**Calc. c.** Leucorrhœa, with milk - like discharge during micturition, or flowing only by spells. Too early and too profuse menstruation. Very weakly in general, walking produces great fatigue. * Very sensitive to cold air. * Feet feel as if they had on cold damp stockings. Scrofulous diathesis.

**China.** Weakly persons who have lost much blood. * Leucorrhœa before the menses, with painful pressing towards the groins and anus. * Bloody leucorrhœa, with occasional discharge of black clots, or fetid purulent matter. Troublesome itching and spasmodic contraction in the inner parts.

**Cocc.** Scanty irregular menses, with leucorrhœa between the periods. * Discharge like serum, mixed with a purulent, ichorous liquid. * When bending or sitting down the discharge escapes in a gush. Painful menstruation followed by hemorrhoids. Abdomen distended, with sharp, cutting pains, worse by motion.

**Coni.** Weakness and lameness in the small of the back. * Leucorrhœa, smarting, and excoriating the parts. Discharge whitish or milk-colored and painful. Induration or ulceration of the os uteri. * Vertigo during the menses, particularly while lying down. Dysmenorrhœa, with shooting pain in the left side of the chest.

**Graph.** Females inclined to obesity; menses too *late* and too *scanty*. * *Leucorrhœa profuse* and of a white color. Great weakness in the small of the back when walking or sitting. * Eruptions on the skin oozing out a sticky fluid.

**Igna.** Violent labor-like pains, with pressing in the region of the womb. * Purulent, corrosive leucorrhœa, with a weak empty feeling in the stomach. * She seems full of suppressed grief. Difficult stools causing prolapsus ani.

**Kali bi.** * Yellow, ropy leucorrhœa, which can be *drawn out in long strings.* Much pain and weakness across the small of the back. Menses too soon, with vertigo, nausea, and headache.

**Kreosot.** Leucorrhœa *before* and after the menses. * Putrid, acrid, corrosive leucorrhœa, with great debility, particularly of the lower extremities. Menses too early, too profuse, and last too long. * She always feels chilly at the menstrual period.

**Lach.** Leucorrhœa before the menses. * Discharge copious, smarting, slimy, stiffening the linen and staining it green. Menses regular, but too short and feeble. * Inability to bear anything tight around the waist. Women at the *critical age.*

**Lyc.** * Profuse leucorrhœa at intervals, accompanied by a *cutting pain across* the *hypogastrium* from *right* to *left.* Pale face, with frequent flushes or circumscribed redness of the cheeks. * Red sandy sediment in the urine. Menses too long and too profuse. * Sense of great fulness in the stomach, after eating ever so little.

**Nux v.** Fetid leucorrhœa tingeing the linen yellow, with pain in the uterus as if sprained. * Menses irregular, never at the right time. Habitual constipation, with frequent urging to stool. As a consequence of high living, or of a sedentary life.

**Podo.** Leucorrhœa, attended with constipation, and bearing down in the genital organs. Discharge consisting of thick transparent mucus. * Prolapsus uteri and ani. *Morning diarrhœa;* stools watery and green.

**Puls.** Burning, thin, acrid leucorrhœa. * Milky leucorrhœa, with swelling of the vulva, particularly after the menses. Also, leucorrhœa with thick white mucus before and during the menses. * Vertigo when rising from a sitting posture, with chilliness. *Mild, tearful* women.

**Sepia**. Climacteric period, during pregnancy or puberty. Leucorrhœa with stitches in the neck of the uterus, and itching in the vagina. Yellowish, watery, milk-like, or mucous leucorrhœa. * Dirty yellow spots on the face. Very fetid urine, depositing a clay-colored sediment.

**Sulph.** Burning and painful leucorrhœa, making the vulva sore. Discharge thin, yellowish, preceded by pinching in the hypogastrium. * Burning in the vagina. * Frequent weak, faint spells during the day. * Constant heat on top of the head. Burning in the soles of the feet; puts them out of bed to get cool.

---

## MEASLES.

**Therapeutics.** Special indications.

**Acon.** At the beginning, when there is dry and hot skin, full, quick pulse and much thirst. * Eyes red, watery, and sensitive to light. Catarrhal irritation, with dry hacking, or hoarse, croupy cough. * Great anxiety and restlessness. Headache, and vertigo on rising up.

**Apis.** Confluent eruption and œdematous swelling of the skin. * Cough and soreness in the chest as if bruised. Oppression of the chest, with inability to remain in a warm room. Scanty and high-colored urine. * Diarrhœa in the morning, stools greenish-yellow.

**Ars.** In severe cases, when typhoid symptoms are present. * Burning and great dryness and itching of the skin. The eruption disappears too suddenly. * Bloatedness of the face, and dry, parched lips. * Great anguish, restlessness, and fear of death. * Constant craving for cold water, drinking often but little at a time. *Rapid prostration.* Aggravation about midnight.

**Bell.** Bright-red appearance of the throat and

tongue, with difficulty of swallowing. * Red and hot face, with throbbing headache. Feeling in the back as if it would break. Dry, spasmodic cough. Constant drowsiness, and moaning during sleep. * Starting and jumping during sleep, with flushed face and red eyes. If *complicated with scarlet fever.*

**Bry.** The eruption is imperfectly developed. * Congestion of the chest, with shooting, stitching pains, increased by deep breathing. * Great dyspnœa and quick breathing. Dry, painful cough, with roughness and dryness of the larynx. * Sitting up in bed causes nausea and faintness. Thirst for large draughts of water.

**Camph.** When there seems to be a depression of the vital forces. * Face pale, and the skin cold, assuming a bluish color. * The eruption does not make its appearance as it should. Great prostration and spasmodic stiffness of the body. * Coldness of the skin, yet the patient cannot bear to be covered.

**Coff.** Measly spots on the skin, with dry heat at night. * Great sensitiveness, with general excitability. * Extreme wakefulness. Dry, hacking cough, with constant tickling in the larynx.

**Ipec.** Eruption slow to make its appearance, with oppression of the chest. * Constant tickling cough with every breath, and rattling of phlegm in the chest. * Much nausea and vomiting. *Suppression of the eruption.* Constant sense of nausea.

**Merc.** The glands of the throat are much swollen, and there is difficulty in swallowing. * Soreness of the throat and *ulceration* of the tonsils. Profuse secretion of saliva, and bad breath. * Great sensitiveness of the pit of the stomach. Much perspiration without relief. Diarrhœa, with green, slimy, or bloody stools, with *severe tenesmus.*

**Phos.** If the disease be complicated with pneumonia, or if typhoid symptoms set in. * Tightness across the chest, with violent and exhausting cough and *rust-colored* sputa. Sticking pains in the chest, aggravated by coughing or breathing. * Hoarseness, with loss of voice.

**Puls.** Generally in the beginning, when the catarrhal symptoms first appear. Eyes red, watery and sensitive to light. Thick, yellow discharge from the nose. * Dryness of the mouth without thirst. * The eruption is tardy in coming out. Loose cough, with thick, yellow mucous expectoration. * Nightly diarrhœa. * Craves cool, fresh air, worse in a warm room. Increase of all the symptoms towards evening.

---

## MENORRHAGIA.

**Therapeutics.** Special indications.

**Acon.** Adapted to plethoric females and lively young girls. * Profuse menses, with great fear and anxiety of mind. * Vertigo on rising from a recumbent position. If induced by exposure to a dry, cold wind.

**Amm. c.** Premature and profuse menstruation, with spasmodic pain. Discharge *blackish* or *light-colored;* acrid, making the thighs sore. Great sadness, and pain in the small of the back.

**Bell.** Too early and too profuse menstruation. Discharge bright red, with coagula having a bad smell. * Violent pressing down as if everything would escape through the genitals. * Throbbing headache, and pain in the small of the back. Clutching pain in the hypogastrium, with screaming, and disposition to bite and tear things.

**Bry.** Too early and too profuse. * Discharge dark-red, with lacerating pains in the limbs. Pain in the back, and headache as if the skull would split open. Cannot sit up on account of nausea and faintness. * Wants to remain quiet and still, the least motion makes her worse. * Constipation, stools hard and dry as if burnt. Very *irritable,* everything makes her angry. Lips dry and cracked.

**Calc. c.** Menstruation too soon, too profuse, and lasting too long. Preceding the flow, there is swelling and sensitiveness of the breasts, headache, colic, and shiverings. During the flow, cutting in the abdomen, toothache and bearing down. * Vertigo when stooping, worse on rising or going up-stairs. * Feet feel as if they had on cold, damp stockings. Very *sensitive to the least cold air.*

**Calc. phos.** Menses every two weeks, black and clotted. Preceding the flow, griping and rumbling in the bowels. Stitching pains in the left side of the head. Sleepiness during the day.

**Cham.** * Profuse discharge of dark and clotted blood, flowing at intervals. * Violent labor-like pains in the uterus, and tearing in the veins of the legs. Very *impatient*, can hardly answer a civil question. Frequent desire to pass urine.

**Cimicifu.** Too early and profuse. Discharge dark and coagulated. * Severe pain in the back and down the thighs. Aching across the hips, and pressing down in the uterus. Great nervousness, and hysterical spasms. Severe pain in the head and eyeballs, increased by the least motion.

**Croc.** Menses regular, but too *profuse* and long-continued. * Discharge dark, clotted, stringy blood. * The least movement increases the flow. Yellowish earthy color of the face. * Sensation as of something moving in the abdomen. Great debility and palpitation of the heart on going up-stairs.

**Igna.** Too frequent, profuse, and long-lasting. * The patient seems full of suppressed grief. * Frequent involuntary sighing, with a feeling of emptiness in the stomach. Difficult stool causing prolapsus ani. Cold hands and feet; also numbness of the feet and legs.

**Iodine.** Menses premature, copious and violent, with great weakness. Discharge preceded by heat in the head and palpitation of the heart. * Ovarian region painful, or sensitive to pressure. * Emaciation with a *good appetite.* Hard, knotty, dark-colored stools.

**Nux mos.** Menses too early and too profuse, with discharge of *thick, black blood.* * Tongue and mouth very dry, particularly after sleeping. Great pressure in the back from within outwards during the menses. * Drowsiness and inclination to faint. * Pain in the sacrum when riding in a carriage. Great *distention* of the *abdomen after eating.*

**Nux v.** Menses too early and too profuse; discharge dark-colored blood. * The flow after continuing several days, stops and then returns. Dragging about the loins, with bearing down in the pelvis. * Cramp-like pains in the abdomen extending down to the thighs. * She gets angry and violent without provocation. Habitual constipation, with frequent *urging to stool.*

**Phos.** Menses *too soon*, too copious, and lasting *too long*, with pain in the small of the back and in the abdomen. Great weakness, with cold feet and legs. * Sensation of weakness and emptiness in the abdomen. * Belching up large quantities of wind after eating. Very sleepy after meals, especially after dinner. * Long, slim, hard, difficult stools. Tall, slender people, with fair skin.

**Sabina.** *Very profuse* and debilitating menses. Discharge partly pale-red and partly clotted blood. * Labor - like pains drawing down into the groin. * Drawing, tearing pains from the back through to the pubis. Very nervous and hysterical. Great liability to miscarry.

**Secale.** Too profuse and too long continued. Discharge dark, liquid blood, increased by motion. * All her common ailments worse just before the menses. Suitable to thin, scrawny women.

**Sepia.** Mostly too early and profuse. Before the menses, violent colic. * Painful sensation of emptiness at the pit of the stomach. * Fetid urine, having a sediment like burnt clay. *Yellow spots on the face*, especially across the nose. * Prolapsus uteri. * Sensation as if everything would escape through the vagina.

**Sulph.** The menses last too long. * She seems to get almost well, and then it returns again, and again. Discharge acrid, corroding the thighs, and smelling sour. * Flashes of heat, followed by weak, faint spells. * Constant heat on top of the head. Bleeding hemorrhoids.

**Trillium.** Menses lasting too long; discharge at

first bright-red, but grows pale. Between the periods, profuse leucorrhœa of a yellowish color and creamy consistence. Profuse hemorrhages.

---

## METRITIS.

**Therapeutics.** Special indications.

**Acon.** After a violent chill; dry, hot skin, full bounding pulse, and intense thirst. Cutting, lancinating, burning, and tearing pains in the region of the uterus, with anguish and great fear. Suppression of the lochia, or too scanty discharge. * Excessive sensibility to the least touch. * Retention of urine, with stitches in the kidneys. * Fear of death, predicts the day she will die. Great restlessness and nervous excitability.

**Arnica.** If the disease was induced by *external violence, as a blow or concussion.* * Sore bruised feeling all through the body. * The bed on which she lies feels too hard, which makes her constantly change about. Putrid eructations.

**Ars.** Mostly in the advanced stages. Burning, lancinating pains; the parts *burn like fire.* * Great anguish, extreme restlessness and fear of death. *Rapid prostration,* with sinking of the vital forces. * Craves cold drinks, but can take but little at a time. Wants to be covered up warmly. Aggravation at night, particularly after midnight.

**Bell.** Great tenderness of the abdomen, aggravated by the least jar, even of the bed. * Violent clutching pains, as if the parts were seized with *talons* (clawing). * Pains come on suddenly and cease as suddenly as they come. Great *heat* in the abdomen, which imparts a *burning* sensation to the hand. * Almost constant moaning, with starting and jumping while sleeping. Painful bearing down in the pelvis. Suppression of the lochial or menstrual discharge, or else it is scant and fetid. Congestion to the head, with flushed face and red eyes. Throbbing headache, and also delirium. * Great intolerance to light or noise.

**Bry.** Stitching, burning pains in the abdomen, which is tender to touch. * Lochia *suppressed*, with headache as if it would split open. Lips parched, dry, and cracked. Great dryness of the mouth, with little thirst, or else drinking large quantities. * Cannot sit up from nausea and faintness. * Wants to remain perfectly quiet; worse from the least motion. * Constipation of hard, dry stools as if burnt. Exceedingly irritable.

**Canth.** Great heat and burning in the abdomen. Debility, restlessness, and trembling of the limbs. * Constant, painful urging and tenesmus of the bladder, passing but a few drops at a time, sometimes mixed with blood.

**Cham.** If the disease was induced by a fit of anger. Heat all over, with thirst and red face, or *one cheek is red and the other pale.* * Violent labor-like pains in the uterus. *Profuse lochia.* Great sensitiveness to pain, becomes almost furious. * She is very impatient, can hardly answer a civil question. Urine abundant and light-colored. Warm sweat about the head.

**Colo.** * Terrible colicky pains, causing her to bend double, with great restlessness. * Feeling in the abdomen as if the intestines were being squeezed between stones. Vomiting and diarrhœa, worse after eating or drinking. Bitter taste in the mouth. Full, frequent pulse, and great thirst.

**Hyos.** If the disease assume a typhoid character. * Spasmodic jerking of the limbs, face, and eyelids. Furious delirium, with wild, staring look. * Muttering, and picking at the bed-clothes. * She throws off the bed-clothes and wants to be naked. Complete apathy, or else great excitability.

**Ipec.** Pain in the region of the umbilicus, extending towards the uterus. Every movement is attended with a cutting pain, running from *left to right.* * Continual nausea and vomiting. Discharge from the womb of bright-red blood. * Green, watery, fermented stools.

**Lach.** * Cannot bear any pressure, not even the clothing over the uterine region. * The pain in the uterus is relieved for a time by a flow of blood, but soon returns. Repeated chills, livid face and unconsciousness. Skin alternately hot and cold. Abdomen distended. Lochial discharge thin and ichorous. * Aggravation after sleep.

**Merc.** Lancinating, boring or pressing pains in the genital organs. * Very sensitive about the pit of the stomach and abdomen. Much saliva in the mouth. * Tongue moist, with great thirst. Much perspiration, which affords no relief. Aggravation at night. * Green, slimy, or bloody mucous stools with violent tenesmus.

**Nux v.** Feeling of heaviness and burning in the genital organs and abdomen. Suppression, or else too profuse discharge of the lochia, with violent pains in the small of the back. Pain as if bruised in the neck of the uterus. * Constipation, with frequent and ineffectual urging to stool. Pain in the small of the back, much worse when attempting to turn in bed. Aggravation in the morning.

**Puls.** After taking cold, particularly after getting the feet wet. * Frequent chilliness, even in a warm room. Inflammation of the uterus, with suppression of the lochial or menstrual discharge. Contractive or labor-like pains in the uterus. Semi-lateral headache. Nightly diarrhœa. * Thirstlessness, and bad taste in the mouth. Mild, tearful persons.

**Rhus t.** Metritis after confinement. * She cannot lie still, but must change continually to get a little rest. * The lower limbs seem powerless, she can hardly draw them up. Dry tongue with red tip. Typhoid symptoms. Aggravation *during rest*, at night, particularly after midnight.

**Secale.** Tendency to putrescence. Hot fever, intermingled by shaking chills. Discharge from the vagina of thin black blood, very offensive. Great anguish, pain in the pit of the stomach, and vomiting of decomposed matters. Painless diarrhœa, with much debility. She lies either in quiet delirium, or grows wild with great anxiety and desire to escape from bed. * Thin, scrawny women. * Desire to be uncovered.

**Stram.** Face red and bloated. Extreme degree of nervous erethism. Convulsive trembling and restlessness. * She awakens with a shrinking look, as if afraid of the first object seen. Talks continually, and imagines all sorts of absurd things.

**Verat. alb.** Puerperal metritis, with violent fits *of vomiting and diarrhœa.* *Coldness of the extremities, with deadly-pale face, covered with cold perspiration. Suppression of the lochial discharge, with delirium. *Excessive weakness.

---

## METRORRHAGIA.

**Therapeutics.** Special indications.

**Acon.** In persons of a full plethoric habit, especially young girls. * Active hemorrhage, with fear of death and great nervous excitability. So giddy, she cannot sit up in bed.

**Bell.** Pale or flushed face. Violent pains in small of the back, as if it would break. * Profuse discharge of bright-red, hot blood, with violent pressure downward as if everything would escape through the vulva. The blood sometimes has a bad smell. Palpitation of the heart.

**Bry.** Discharge of dark-red blood in large quantities, with violent pressive pains in small of the back, and headache as if it would split. * Nausea and faintness on sitting up in bed. Mouth and lips unusually dry with thirst. *Symptoms all worse by moving; she wants to keep perfectly quiet. Exceedingly irritable. Dry, hard stools.

**Cham.** Hemorrhage of dark, coagulated blood, with *labor-like pains.* Tearing pains in the legs. Frequent discharge of large quantities of colorless urine. *Very impatient; can hardly give one a civil answer.

**China.** After miscarriage or labor, and in dangerous cases. Discharge of clots of dark blood. * Heaviness of the head, ringing in the ears, loss of sight, and fainting. Sudden weakness, coldness of the extremities, and pale face. Colic, frequent urging to urinate, and sore tension in the abdomen. *Debility and other troubles after the loss of much blood.

**Croc.** After miscarriage or labor, or from over-exertion. *Discharge of dark, stringy blood, worse from the least exertion. Sensation as of something rolling or moving about in the abdomen. Passive hemorrhage, in nervous, hysterical women.

**Ferr. m.** Weakly persons of hemorrhagic tendency Frequent discharge of partly fluid and partly black clotted blood, with violent labor-like pains. *The least emotion or exertion produces a red flushed face Frequent short shudderings; headache and vertigo.

**Hyos.** Flooding attended with labor-like pains in the uterus, drawing in the thighs and small of the back. Bright-red blood continuing to flow all the time. Heat all over the body, with a quick or full pulse. Trembling over the whole body, or numbness of the limbs. *Twitching or jerking of single limbs

**Ipec.** *Very copious flooding of bright-red blood coming away in a gush, with cutting pains around the navel. Great pressure and bearing down. Chills and coldness of the body. Great weakness and inclination to vomit. After *parturition or miscarriage.*

**Sabina.** Forcing or dragging pains extending to the back and loins. Profuse discharge of bright-red blood. Feeling of sinking or faintness in the abdomen. *Sometimes the discharge is dark, having blackish clots mixed with thin watery blood. Pains extending from the back through to the pubis.

**Secale.** *Passive hemorrhage in feeble cachectic females. After parturition or miscarriage. Discharge of dark liquid blood, with little or no pain. Coldness of the extremities, pale or sallow face, and small feeble pulse. Desire to be uncovered, worse from warmth.

**Sepia.** Induration of the neck of the uterus, with spasmodic painful pressure over the sexual organs. Chronic metrorrhagia, when it is excited from the least cause. Yellow complexion, with spots on the face. *Painful sense of emptiness in the abdomen. Fetid urine, depositing a clay-colored sediment which adheres to the vessel.

**Sulph.** Frequent attacks of hemorrhage; she seems

to get almost well, when it occurs again and again. * Constant heat in top of the head, and cold feet. Frequent weak faint spells and flushes of heat. Gets very hungry about 11 A. M., cannot wait for dinner.

---

## MISCARRIAGE.

**Therapeutics.** Special indications.

**Acon.** Threatened miscarriage in consequence of fright. * Hemorrhage, with fear of death; she is sure she will die. Great fear and anxiety of mind, with great nervous excitability. Dizziness on rising from a recumbent position. Feverish restlessness.

**Apis.** *Stinging* pains in the ovarian region. Pressing-down, or labor-like pain, in the uterus. * Sensation in the abdomen as if something tight would break, if much effort was made to void a stool. Scanty urine, and absence of thirst. Aggravation in a warm room.

**Arnica.** After a *fall*, *blow*, or *concussion*, especially if labor-pains set in, with discharge of blood or serous mucus. * Sore feeling all through the patient, as if from a bruise. The bed on which she lies feels too hard.

**Bell.** Flushed face, red eyes, throbbing carotids and heat in the head. Pain in the back as if it would break. * Severe bearing down, as if everything would issue through the vulva. Profuse discharge of blood, neither very bright, nor dark-colored. * Pains which come on suddenly, and leave just as suddenly. * Vertigo when stooping, or when rising from a stooping posture. Great intolerance to light or noise.

**Calc. c.** Scrofulous diathesis. She has heretofore suffered from too early and too profuse menstruation. She is very weakly in general; walking produces great fatigue, and she is out of breath when going up stairs. When standing, a pressing down, as if everything would come out through the genitals. * Her feet feel as if they had on cold, damp stockings. * Vertigo when ascending a height.

**Cham.** Periodical pains resembling those of *labor*, with discharge of dark-colored or coagulated blood. * Violent pains in the bowels, extending to the sides, with *frequent urination.* Becomes almost furious about the pains. * Very impatient, can hardly answer a civil question. Hot perspiration about the head.

**China.** In weak and exhausted persons from loss of animal fluids. After miscarriage when there is hemorrhage unto fainting; giddiness, drowsiness, and loss of consciousness. * Heaviness of the head, ringing in the ears, and coldness of the extremities. Twitching and jerking of single muscles.

**Croc.** Especially where the discharge consists of *dark, stringy blood, which is increased by the least exertion.* * Sensation of fluttering, or as if something were moving about in the abdomen. Mostly after miscarriage.

**Ferr. m.** After miscarriage, when there is a discharge of partly fluid and partly black, clotted blood, with violent labor-like pains. Full, hard pulse, and short shudderings. * Least emotion or exertion produces a red, flushed face. General hemorrhagic tendency.

**Hyos.** Miscarriage attended with spasms or convulsions of the whole body. Discharge of light-red blood, with labor-like pains. * Twitching and jerking of single muscles or limbs. Adapted to hysterical subjects.

**Igna.** Suppressed grief seems to have been the exciting cause. * Sadness and sighing, with an empty feeling at the pit of the stomach. Uterine cramps with cutting stitches. * Difficult stools causing prolapsus ani.

**Ipec.** * Profuse and continuous discharge of bright-red blood, accompanied with pressure downward. Cutting pains around the navel. * Continual sense of nausea, without a moment's relief. Disposition to faint.

**Nux mos.** Adapted to hysterical females. Pressure in the abdomen, and drawing down into the legs from the navel; discharge *dark and thick.* * Great drowsiness and inclination to faint.

**Nux v.** Every pain produces a desire to go to stool, or to urinate. Much pain in small of the back, which is made worse by turning in bed. Writhing pains in the abdomen, accompanied by nausea, or pains in the back and loins as if dislocated. * Very irritable, and wishes to be alone. Constipation of large difficult stools. Persons who live on rich and highly seasoned food, and live too sedentary.

**Puls.** Labor-like pains alternating with hemorrhage; restlessness. * The discharge is arrested for a little while, then returns with redoubled violence. Suffocative spells; she craves fresh air, and is worse in a close, warm room. * Inclination to be chilly, even in a warm room. Mild, tearful women.

**Rhus t.** * If a wrench or a strain is the exciting cause. Pains worse in the latter part of the night and during rest; has to change position often to get a little temporary relief.

**Sabina.** Violent forcing or dragging pains extending from the *back through to the pubis.* * Discharge profuse, consisting of bright-red, partly fluid and partly-clotted blood. Feeling of sinking or faintness in the abdomen. Especially adapted to women who habitually miscarry about the third month.

**Secale.** Especially after miscarriage has occurred. * Copious flow of black, liquid blood, worse from the slightest motion. * Passive hemorrhage in thin, scrawny, cachectic women. Great debility, feeble almost extinct pulse, and fear of death. Little or no pain.

**Sepia.** Painful sensation of emptiness at the pit of the stomach. * Sense of weight in the anus like a heavy ball. * Yellow saddle across the bridge of the nose. Pressing in the uterus, with oppressed breathing. Very *fetid urine* depositing a clay-colored sediment, which adheres to the vessel with great tenacity.

---

## MORNING SICKNESS.

**Therapeutics.** Special indications.

**Ant. c.** Eructations tasting of the ingesta. Nausea with vertigo. * Frightful and persistent vomiting, with convulsions. Derangement caused by overloading the stomach.

**Arsen.** Excessive vomiting, especially after eating or drinking. * Great desire for water, but can take only a little. * Vomiting of fluids as soon as taken. Great weakness and emaciation; exhausting diarrhœa.

**Bry.** Nausea immediately on waking in the morning. Lips dry and parched; dry mouth and tongue, with much thirst. Vomiting of food immediately after eating it. Headache as if it would split open. * She feels better by keeping perfectly quiet. * Dry, hard stools, as if burnt. Very irritable.

**Calc. c.** Heartburn and eructations of food. Soreness of the sides or tip of the tongue, so that she can scarcely talk or eat. * Going up stairs puts her out of breath; also causes vertigo. * Cold, damp feet continually. Cannot bear tight clothing around the waist. * She cannot sleep after three in the morning.

**Cocc.** Cardialgia after a meal. In the morning, she can scarcely rise up on account of nausea and inclination to vomit; it makes her so faint. * Nausea from riding in a carriage or in a boat.

**Coni.** Terrible nausea and vomiting during pregnancy. Sour eructations, with burning in the stomach. * Vertigo, particularly when lying down and when turning over in bed. Swelling and soreness of the breasts.

**Cyclamen.** After eating the least quantity, disgust and nausea in the palate and throat. Much dimness of vision, with fiery specks and sparks before the eyes. Intermittent thirst.

**Ipec.** Nausea and vomiting, with great uneasiness in the stomach. * Continual nausea all the time, not a moment's relief. * Vomiting of large quantities of mucus. Bilious vomiting, and tendency to relaxation of the bowels.

**Natr. m.** In obstinate cases, accompanied by loss of appetite and taste. Waterbrash, like limpid mucus, and much acidity of the stomach. * Always awakens in the morning with headache, and has heartburn after eating. * Feeling of grèat hunger, as if the stomach were empty, but no appetite.

**Nitric acid.** * Much nausea and gastric trouble, relieved by moving about or riding in a carriage. Constant nausea, with heat in the stomach extending to the throat. *Strong-smelling urine.*

**Nux v.** Nausea and vomiting chiefly in the morning, while eating, or immediately after eating or drinking. Acrid and bitter eructations and regurgitations. * She feels as if she would be better if she could vomit. * Cannot bear the odor of tobacco. Females of sedentary habits, and who are accustomed to the use of highly seasoned food. * Large, difficult stools, with frequent urging.

**Phos.** Nausea with hunger, early in the morning. Very weak feeling in the abdomen, and heat up the back. Sour vomiting and sour eructations. * Long, narrow, hard stools, very difficult to expel. * Very sleepy after meals, particularly after dinner.

**Puls.** Frequent eructations, tasting of the ingesta. Vomiting after every meal. * Vomiting of mucus. * Bad taste in the mouth every morning on waking. No kind of food tastes good to her. Perceptible pulsations in the pit of the stomach. Diarrhœa, mostly at night. Persons of a mild, tearful disposition.

**Sepia.** Nausea in the morning as if all the viscera were turning inside out. * Sense of emptiness at the pit of the stomach. The very thought of food sickens her. Yellowness of the face, particularly across the nose. Painful feeling of hunger in the stomach.

---

## MUMPS.

**Therapeutics.** Special indications.

**Bell.** Redness of the face and eyes. * Bright-red swelling of the glands, especially on the right side. Tendency to erysipelatous inflammation of the parts affected. * Sudden disappearance of the swelling, with throbbing headache and delirium. * Sleepiness, but cannot sleep.

**Carb. v.** Slow grade of fever; the swelling becomes very hard and will not disperse as it should. * Metastasis to the stomach, with burning, pressure and sensitiveness of the epigastrium. After abuse of calomel. * The most innocent food disagrees. Much belching of sour, rancid food.

**Hyos.** If the disease be transmitted to the brain. Unconscious delirium, red face, wild, staring look, and throbbing of the carotids. * Twitching and jerking of the limbs, with great nervous excitability. Giddiness, with stupefaction.

**Merc.** If the disease was induced by a cold. Erethic fever, with alternate heat and chills. Hard swelling of the gland, with stiffness of the jaws and difficulty of swallowing. Thirst, particularly at night. * Perspiration, affording no relief. * Profuse secretion of saliva, and very offensive breath. Dark-green or slimy stools with *severe tenesmus.* All worse at night, and in damp rainy weather.

**Puls.** When there is metastasis to the female mammæ, or to the testicles of the male. Inflammation and swelling of the testicles, with drawing pain extending up the spermatic cords. * Vertigo when rising from a sitting posture, with chilliness. * Thickly-coated tongue, with very bad taste in the morning. Mild, tearful disposition.

**Rhus t.** If typhoid symptoms set in, or the inflammation assumes an erysipelatous character. Lameness and stiffness of the limbs, with pain on *first moving them after rest.* * Parotitis after scarlatina, with dropsical symptoms. * Restless at night; must turn often to find a few moments' ease.

---

## NEPHRITIS.

**Therapeutics.** Special indications.

**Acon.** In the early stage, when there is high fever, evinced by hot, dry skin, quick pulse, and intense thirst. * Retention of urine, with stitches in the kidneys. * Fear and anxiety of mind, with great nervous excitability. * So giddy, cannot sit up in bed.

**Bell.** Shooting pains from the kidneys to the bladder. * Pains which appear and disappear suddenly. * Sensation as of a worm writhing in the bladder. Urine scanty, of a bright-red or yellowish color, depositing a whitish thick sediment. Heat and swelling in the region of the kidney. * Back feels as if it would break, hindering motion. Throbbing pain in the forehead.

**Cannabis.** Inflammation of the kidneys, with dragging or shooting pains along the ureters to the groin. Painful urging to urinate, passing only a few drops of bloody, burning urine. Burning *during* and *after* micturition.

**Canth.** Burning heat, with thirst and anxiety. Shooting, cutting, or tearing pains in the loins and region of the kidney. * Constant desire to urinate, passing but a few drops at a time, sometimes mixed with blood. Burning, cutting pains in the bladder, with ineffectual efforts to urinate. * Vomiting, with violent retching and severe colic.

**Hepar.** Where suppuration has occurred, or the formation of abscess is imminent. * Sensation of throbbing in the region of the kidney. Feeling of weight in the loins. Alternate chilliness and heat, followed by profuse perspiration.

**Merc.** For a similar train of symptoms as are described under **Hepar.**, and where that remedy does not produce the desired improvement. Urine scanty and red, with *strong smell.* * Much perspiration, affording no relief.

**Lyc.** * Renal colic, when the pain is felt along the ureters into the bladder, especially on the right side. * Red *sandy* sediment in the urine. Cutting pain across the hypogastrium, from right to left. * Terrific pain in the back previous to every urination, with relief as soon as the urine begins to flow.

**Nux v.** In persons of sedentary habits, or where the disease arises from suppressed hemorrhoids. Pain in small of the back, so bad, he cannot move. * Painful desire to urinate, with scanty emissions in drops, with burning, tearing pains. Reddish urine, with brick-dust-like sediment. * Constipation of hard difficult stools, and frequent urging.

**Puls.** Persons of a mild, tearful disposition, or females with scanty or suppressed menses. Aching pain in small of the back. * Frequent and almost ineffectual urging to urinate, with cutting pain. Chilliness even in a warm room Headache, relieved by compression. *Craves cool fresh air, worse in a warm room. *Bad taste in the morning.* * Vertigo when rising from a sitting posture. Pale watery urine, jelly-like sediment.

**Sepia.** * Yellowness of the face, particularly across the bridge of the nose resembling a saddle. Great sense of emptiness at the pit of the stomach. Intense burning and cutting pain when urinating. * *Fetid urine,* depositing a clay-colored sediment, which adheres to the vessel as if it had been burnt on. * Sense of great weight in the anus, not relieved by stool.

**Sulph.** In chronic or protracted cases where only partial relief has been obtained by other remedies. * Burning and drawing pain in small of the back. Pulsative stitches in the region of the loins and kidneys. Painful desire to urinate, with discharge of drops of bloody urine. * *Very fetid urine.* Frequent weak, faint spell. * Constant heat on top of the head.

**Terebinth.** Burning, drawing pains in the kidneys. Pressure in the bladder, extending up into the kidneys when sitting, disappearing when walking about. * Difficult urination, with burning in the bladder. * Blood is thoroughly mixed with the urine, like coffee-grounds sediment.

Nephritis arising from the use of Spanish fly-blister, will be relieved by **Camphor** in drop-doses.

---

## NEURALGIA.

**Therapeutics.** Special indications.

**Acon.** Red and hot face, with pain on one side. * Pains so severe, the patient becomes desperate, and declares that *something must be done.* * Great fear and anxiety, with vertigo on rising from a sitting posture. Pains worst at night, with great restlessness.

**Ars.** Attacks return periodically, and are chiefly felt around the eye and in the temples. * Burning, stinging pain, as if pierced with red-hot needles. Pain so great at times, as to almost drive one distracted. Great fear and anxiety of mind, with extreme restlessness. Aggravation about midnight. Temporary relief from external heat, and from moving about. Great *prostration.*

**Bell.** Pain most violent under the eye, excited by rubbing the part. * Darting pains in the cheek-bones, nose, or zygomatic process. Cutting and tearing pains, with stiffness at the nape of the neck, and clenching of the jaws. * Violent shooting or tearing pains in the ball of the eye. * Convulsive jerkings in the facial muscles. * Great intolerance to *noise* or *light.* Aggravation in the afternoon.

**Caust.** Tensive or beating pains in the facial bones, especially under the eye. * Drawing pains, mostly on the right side, from the cheek-bone to the temple. Obstinate constipation and hemorrhoids. * Involuntary urination when coughing.

**Cham.** Stitching or jerking pains, that seem intolerable, especially at night. * The pain causes hot perspiration about the head, and extorts cries. * Very impatient, can hardly answer a civil question. Great sensitiveness to pain, becomes almost furious.

**China.** *Periodical attacks.* * Darting, tearing pains, aggravated by the *least contact.* Pain mostly in the infra-orbital and maxillary nerves. * Exacerbation every other day. Weakly persons who have lost much blood.

**Cimicifu.** Intense and persistent pains in the eyeballs, of a dull, aching, sore nature. Sensation as if the top of the head would fly off; the cerebrum feels too large for the skull, pressing outwards and upwards.

**Colo.** Neuralgia chiefly on the left side of the face. * Violent rending and darting pains, aggravated by *touch or motion.* Tearing, screwing pains, together with great restlessness and anxiety. Better from perfect rest, and from warm applications. If caused by anger.

**Gels.** *Throbbing pain in the medulla* passing through the mastoid to the forehead and eyes. Great heaviness of the eyelids, it is impossible to keep them open. Dimness of vision, and confusion of mind.

**Hepar.** Pains in the malar bones, extending to the ears and temples. Worse when in the open air, and better from wrapping up the face. Fluent coryza, with hoarseness and much sweating. After the abuse of mercury.

**Iris v.** Neuralgia of the head, eyes, and temples. * Sharp, cutting pains of short duration, with vomiting of a sweetish mucus. *Burning distress in the epigastrium.* Profuse flow of saliva. Pains aggravated by rest.

**Merc.** Tearing pains, worse at night in bed. * Pain starts in a decayed tooth, and involves the whole side of the face, which may be red and swollen. Profuse ptyalism and lachrymation. * Much perspiration affording no relief. If arisen from a cold.

**Mez.** Chiefly on the left side of the face. The pains extend to the eye, temple, ear, neck, and shoulder. * Boring, pressing pains, coming like lightning, leaving the parts numb. Aggravated by taking warm food or drink, or from entering a warm room after being in the open air.

**Nux v.** Drawing, tearing, or compressive pains, chiefly in the forehead or in the part just above the root of the nose. * Tearing pain in the facial and infra-orbital nerves. Numbness of the affected part. Redness and lachrymation of the eyes. Fluent watery discharge from the nose. Constipation, with frequent urging to stool. * Very irritable, and wishes to be alone. Aggravation in the morning, and from mental exertion.

**Phos.** Drawing and tearing pain in the jaws, root of the nose, eyes, and temples. Face swollen and pale. Vertigo, and buzzing in the ears. * Sensation of weakness and emptiness in the abdomen. * Long, narrow, hard stools, very difficult to expel. Aggravation from chewing, talking, or touching the affected parts.

**Platina.** Severe spasmodic or boring pain in the cheek-bones, with a sensation of crawling or creeping in the parts. * The attack is preceded by a feeling of coldness and torpor. Anxiety, weeping, and palpitation of the heart. Redness of the face and lachrymation. Aggravation in the evening and when at rest.

**Puls.** Mostly on the right side of the face and head. * Darting, tearing pains extending from the jaw to the orbit and temple. * Profuse lachrymation from the affected eye. Chilliness even in a warm room. *Mild, tearful disposition.* Aggravation towards evening and in a warm room. Better from cold, and worse from warm applications.

**Rhus t.** Drawing, burning, tearing pain in the malar bones, root of the nose and ear. * Pain aggravated by rest, must move about continually to get a little relief. Worse at night, particularly after midnight.

**Sepia.** Drawing or cramp-like pains in the facial bones, mostly on the left side. Great sense of emptiness at the pit of the stomach. * Yellowness of the face, particularly across the bridge of the nose resembling a saddle. * Sense of great weight in the anus, not relieved by stool. Especially during the period of gestation.

**Spig.** Periodical neuralgia, mostly on the left side. * Pains darting or burning, especially in the cheekbones, eyeballs, and above the eye. Redness of the parts affected. Flow of water from the eyes and nose. Twitching of the muscles in the face. Palpitation of the heart, and difficulty of breathing. * Pains aggravated by the least contact or motion.

**Staph.** The pain starts in a decayed tooth and extends to the eye. *Drawing*, tearing pains in the cheekbones. Is very sensitive to the least impression. Cold hands and cold sweat in the face. * Pains worse from slight and better from hard pressure.

**Stram.** Many nervous symptoms. * Pains unbearable, driving the patient to despair. Extreme degree of nervous erethism, with convulsive twitching of the muscles of the face. Jerking through the whole body. * Delirious, talking continually; eyes wide open. * Vertigo when walking in the dark.

**Sulph.** Mostly in chronic cases, or where well chosen remedies do not have the desired effect. * After suppressed cutaneous eruptions. Dry, husky, scaly skin; no perspiration. * Constant heat on top of the head. Frequent weak, faint spells.

**Verat. a.** Drawing, tearing pain in the right side of the face and above the ear. Bluish paleness of the face. Sunken eyes and coldness of the extremities. * Attacks of pain, with delirium, or driving to madness. Trembling and jerking of the limbs. * Cold sweat, especially on the forehead.

**Verbascum.** Violent pain jerking like lightning, or pressive numbing. The pain is excited by pressure, sneezing, talking, chewing, etc. Attacks recur at the same hour every day, and is attended with headache, vertigo, belching, and a discharge of tough saliva from the mouth.

**Zinc.** Burning, quick stitches, and jerking along the course of the infra-orbital nerve, right side. Bluish color of the eyelids and numbness of the tongue. Constricted sensation in the throat. * Constant trembling of the hands, with coldness of the extremities. * Fidgety feeling in the feet, must move them constantly.

---

## OPHTHALMIA.

**Therapeutics.** Special indications.

**Acon.** Purulent ophthalmia, where the inflammation runs high; dry, hot skin and full, quick pulse. * Intense redness and swelling of the affected parts, attended with acute pain. *Great intolerance to light.* * Fear, anxiety, and great restlessness. Flushed cheeks, and throbbing of the arteries about the neck.

**Ars.** Inflammation of the conjunctiva and sclerotica, with *dark redness and congestion of the vessels*

* Burning pains; the parts burn like fire. Inflammatory swelling of the lids. Specks or ulcers on the cornea. * Nightly agglutination of the lids. *Great anguish and restlessness.* * Intense thirst, drinking little and often.

**Calc. c.** * Scrofulous ophthalmia. Inflammation, redness, and purulent secretion from the eyeballs. * Swelling and redness of the eyelids, with nightly agglutination. * Stinging pains, worse from candle-light. Specks and ulcers on the cornea. Constant desire to keep the eyes in darkness. Glandular swellings of the neck, and eruptions on the hairy scalp.

**Bell.** Acute ophthalmia, *with very great intolerance to light or noise.* * Vivid redness of the sclerotica, with discharge of hot, salt tears, or great dryness of the eyes. Sharp pains in the orbits, extending to the brain. Pains which appear suddenly, and cease as suddenly. Dimness of vision. Throbbing headache, increased by motion.

**Euphr.** Aching pain in the eyes and redness of the sclerotica. Vesicles, or specks and ulcers on the cornea. * Copious secretion of mucus and tears. Swelling of the eyeballs. * Fluent coryza and headache. Photophobia, flickering of the light.

**Graph.** Scrofulous ophthalmia, or chronic congestion of the conjunctiva. Purulent secretion from the balls and lids, with frequent agglutination. Ulcers on the cornea. Eyelids much inflamed and painful. Constant desire to keep the eyes covered. * Unhealthy skin, with eruptions oozing out a *sticky glutinous fluid.*

**Lyc.** Agglutination of the lids at night, and lachrymation by day. * Burning and smarting in the eyes. Scrofulous or catarrhal ophthalmia. Aptness to take cold. * Red sediment like sand in the urine. Obstinate constipation. * Constant sensation of satiety, feels full up to the throat.

**Merc.** *Gonorrhœal,* or *scrofulous* ophthalmia. Violent inflammation and redness of the eyes. * Cutting, burning pains, or pressure in the eyes as if from sand. Excessive sensitiveness of the eyes to the glare of fire, or to the light. * Vesicles and pimples on the sclerotica. Pustules and scurfs around the eyes and on the margins of the lids.

**Nitr. ac.**, and **Hepar.**, are the best remedies for the removal of mercurial ophthalmia, following the abuse of this drug in syphilis and other diseases.

**Puls.** Catarrhal or rheumatic ophthalmia. Pressure and burning in the eyes as if from sand. Redness and swelling of the conjunctiva and lids. Burning and corrosive lachrymation. Itching and burning of the eyes, inducing a disposition to rub them. * Evening aggravation. Mild, tearful disposition.

**Spig.** Rheumatic and arthritic ophthalmia. Pains of a pressive or stitching character, worse from movement. Vessels of the conjunctiva much congested. Upper lids swollen and stiff. * Aching pains deep in the orbits when touched.

**Sulph.** Scrofulous ophthalmia. * Itching and burning in the eyes and eyelids, worse by moving or exposing them to the sunlight. * Feeling as of sand in the eyes. Specks, vesicles, and ulcers on the cornea. * Flashes of heat, and weak, faint spells. * Burning on top of the head. After suppressed cutaneous eruptions.

---

## PERICARDITIS, ETC.

Although Pericarditis, Endocarditis, Myocarditis, and Hypertrophy of the heart, are usually considered under separate heads, yet their cause, and the tissues involved are so intimately connected, that the remedies adapted to one, will be found correspondingly appropriate to the others.

**Therapeutics.** Special indications.

**Acon.** Full bounding pulse, dry burning skin, agonized tossing about, violent thirst, red face, and shortness of breath. * Great fear and anxiety of mind, with great nervous excitability. * Lancinating pain in the chest, hindering respiration. Has to sit straight up, can hardly breathe. * Fear of death, predicts the day he will die.

**Arnica.** If caused by external injuries. Lancinating pain in the region of the heart, causing faintness Oppression of the chest and great difficulty of breathing. * Sore feeling all through the patient as if from a bruise. * The bed on which he lies feels too hard, causing him to change from place to place.

**Ars.** Inflammation consequent upon the suppression of measles, scarlet fever, or the drying up of old sores. *Violent palpitation of the heart,* particularly at night, and when lying down. * Great anguish, extreme restlessness, and *fear of death.* Dyspnœa, cannot lie down for fear of suffocation. *Rapid prostration.* * Extreme thirst, drinks little and often.

**Aspar.** Chronic organic affections of the heart. Throbbing of the heart, perceptible to the hand and ear, setting in after slight motion. * Irregular, quick, double beats of the heart, with anxiety.

**Aurum.** Endocarditis consequent upon previously existing rheumatic affections. Distressing, anxious pains, preventing the patient from lying down. * Has to sit perfectly quiet in an upright position. Irregular intermittent pulse. * Great melancholy, and loathing of life.

**Bry.** Where the disease is complicated with rheumatism or disorders of the pulmonary structure. * Stitching pains in the region of the heart, aggravated by breathing or motion. * Wants to lie perfectly quiet. Intermittent pulse. * Hard, dry stools, as if burnt. Exceedingly irritable, everything makes him angry.

**Cactus.** Acute pains in the region of the heart, and difficulty of breathing. * Feeling of constriction at the heart, as if an *iron band* prevented its normal action. Palpitation worse when walking, and at night when lying on the left side. Attacks of suffocation, with fainting.

**Cann.** Tensive aching pain behind the sternum. Frequent beatings in both sides of the chest, most painful in the region of the heart. Violent shocks in the region of the heart, as if it would fall out, when stooping or making exertion. Sensation of fulness about the heart.

**Dig.** If caused by protracted grief, care, or anxiety. *Sharp stitches, or contractive pains in the region of the heart. Uneasy sensation in the left side of the chest, often extending to the shoulder and arm. *Palpitation excited by talking, motion, or on lying down. Short hurried breathing. *Œdema* of the feet and legs. Bloated, pale face.

**Iod.** Scrofulous subjects. Pressing sensation in the region of the heart. *Violent palpitation, increased from the slightest motion. Better when lying perfectly still on the back. *Extreme weakness and loss of breath on going up stairs. Fainting spells.

**Kali c.** Stitches in the region of the heart, with frequent and violent palpitation. Crampy pain about the heart, as if bands were firmly drawn round it. *A blowing noise, and a louder second tick of the pulmonary artery is heard, *Swelling over the upper eyelids, like little bags, in the morning. Aggravation about 3 A. M.

**Lach.** Constrictive sensation about the heart. Palpitation with much anxiety. Irregularity of the beats of the heart. Sudden oppression of the chest, accompanied by cough and palpitation. *Cannot lie down, must sit up, bent forwards. *Can bear nothing to touch the neck or throat. Aggravation after sleep.

**Phos.** *Tightness across the chest,* with difficulty of breathing and great weakness. Palpitation, worse after eating, or from mental emotion. Congestion of the lungs, tight cough, and spitting of blood. *Constipation of hard, *narrow,* difficult stools, or painless diarrhœa.

**Puls.** Persons of a mild, tearful disposition. Heaviness, pressure, and burning in the region of the heart. Pain in small of the back, and palpitation of the heart. *Loose, rattling cough, worse on first lying down at night. Rheumatic pains, which quickly change locality. Nightly diarrhœa. *Scanty or suppressed menses. All worse *towards evening.*

**Rhus t.** Sensation of weakness and trembling of the heart. Violent palpitation on sitting still. *Stitches in the heart, with painful lameness and numbness of the left arm. *Pains worse during rest, has to change position often to get relief.

**Spig.** Organic disease of the heart. (Rubbing bellows sound.) * Palpitation so violent, it can be seen and heard at a distance. * Can lie only on the right side, with the trunk well raised. The least motion produces great suffocation, anxiety, and palpitation. * Stitching pains in the chest from the slightest motion. Rheumatic pericarditis.

**Sulph.** If caused from suppressed eruptions or hemorrhoidal discharges. Palpitation of the heart, especially when going up stairs, with shortness of breath. Sensation as if the heart was enlarged. Steady pain in the left side through to the shoulders. * Frequent weak, faint spells. * Constant heat on top of the head. * Early morning diarrhœa. Dry, husky, scaly skin. Sleeplessness.

**Verat. alb.** Paroxysms of anguish about the heart, which beats very strongly. Violent, visible, anxious palpitation of the heart. Stitches in the sides of the chest, worse when coughing. * Cold sweat on the forehead. * Exhausting diarrhœa, with great weakness after every stool. Anguish and fear of death. Sensation as of a lump of ice on top of the head.

---

## PERTUSSIS.

**Therapeutics.** Special indications.

**Acon.** If a constant febrile condition prevails, and when at the commencement the cough is dry, whistling, with soreness of the throat. * The child grasps at its throat with every cough as if it were in pain. * Great anguish, restlessness, and anxiety.

**Ambra gris.** Severe paroxysms of hollow-sounding cough, worse morning and evening and during the night. Oppression and rapid respiration. Expectoration of large quantities of tough, grayish or yellow mucus, especially in the morning.

**Anacar.** When fits of anger cause paroxysms of cough, and when children are very ill-natured. Difficulty of breathing accompanies and succeeds the coughing spells. *Children with uncontrollable tempers.

**Arn.** Left cheek swollen and red, with heat in the head and coldness of the body. * Every coughing spell is preceded by crying. Feels sore all over as if bruised. Bleeding from the nose.

**Ars.** Suffocative, dry cough, with scanty or suppressed urine. * Great prostration, with waxy paleness and coldness of the skin. * Intense thirst, drinks little and often. * Feels better in a warm room Aggravation at night, particularly after midnight.

**Bell.** Frequent paroxysms of cough, worse in the night, hard and barking like croup. * The child gets very red in the face with every coughing spell. * Eyes swollen, and the sclerotica injected with blood. *Bleeding of the nose.* In the beginning, or when the disease has attained a high degree of severity.

**Bry.** Paroxysms set in principally in the evening or at night, or after *eating* or *drinking with vomiting.* * Cough with expectoration of brownish phlegm with stitches through the chest. * Constipation, with dry, hard stools, as if burnt. Exceedingly irritable, everything makes him angry. Lips parched, dry, and cracked.

**Carb. v.** Spasmodic hollow cough, with bloody expectoration. * Great exhaustion after every coughing spell, with blueness of the skin, hot head and face. Small rapid pulse and cold sweat. Sensation as if the œsophagus was contracted. * Stomach and bowels greatly distended with flatulence.

**Cham.** Dry cough, worse at night, or in the cold air. * Child very fretful, must be carried all the time to keep it quiet. * One cheek red and hot, and the other pale and cold. Green watery corroding stools, smelling like rotten eggs. * Warm sweat about the head.

**Cina.** * During the paroxysm, the child suddenly becomes stiff. After the paroxysm, there is a gurgling noise from the throat to the abdomen. Cough aggravated by running, talking, laughing, &c. * Paleness of the face and blueness around the mouth and eyes.

Spasms with jerking and twitching of the muscles. * Much picking of the nose, and other worm symptoms.

**Cocus cacti.** Nightly, periodical attacks of cough, from tickling in the larynx. * Every coughing spell ends with expectoration of large quantities of viscid, stringy mucus.

**Coral. rub.** Spasms of cough, so violent that the child *loses* its *breath* and *turns purple* and *black* in the face. * Takes very little food or drink. Spasmodic convulsive cough.

**Cup.** Violent and long-continued paroxysms of cough, completely exhausting the patient. * During the attack, the child becomes rigid, turns black in the face, and seems as if dead. Vomiting after the paroxysm, and rattling of mucus in the chest between the attacks.

**Dros.** The paroxysm is extremely violent, with chills and fever. * Violent spasmodic cough, threatening suffocation. * Worse particularly after twelve at night. Vomiting of food or mucus, and bleeding from the mouth and nose.

**Hepar.** Dry, spasmodic, croupy cough, with soreness of the larynx, worse towards morning. * Cough sounds croupy, and it seems as if the patient would choke. Rattling, choking cough, worse after midnight. * Cannot bear to be uncovered, coughs when any part of the body is exposed.

**Kali bi.** Violent, rattling cough, lasting some minutes, with an effort to vomit. * Choking cough, with expectoration of viscid mucus, which can be drawn out in long strings. Burning pain in the trachea and bronchia.

**Lach.** * The slightest pressure on the larynx produces violent and long-continued cough. * Child always awakens in a coughing fit. Can bear nothing tight about the neck, or waist.

**Merc.** Cough only at night, or only during the day. * Two paroxysms succeed each other closely, and are separated from the next two by an interval of perfect rest. During the vomiting the patient bleeds at the nose and mouth. * Profuse sweat at night, with nervous agitation. Much trouble from ascarides.

**Nux v.** Hard, dry cough, worse in the morning * The child has choking spells, becomes blue in th face, bleeds at the nose and mouth. Gagging, vomit ing and constipation. During the paroxysm, pain i the umbilical region as if it would be torn to pieces After nostrums and cough-mixtures.

**Puls.** Cough from the beginning, with profuse ex pectoration. Frequent vomiting of mucus or the in gesta. Diarrhœa, especially at night. * Chillines even in a warm room, and vertigo on rising from sitting posture. Mild, tearful persons, with blue eye and blonde hair.

**Sulph.** Scrofulous subjects. Frequent relapse without any known cause. Dry, suppressed, chokin cough. Unhealthy skin, dry, husky, and scaly. N sweat from the beginning. * Frequent weak, fain spells. * Much rattling of mucus in the chest. Con stipation, or *morning diarrhœa.*

**Squill.** During the cough the child sneezes, water at the nose and eyes. * Constant rubbing of the nose face, and eyes during the cough. Cough *excited* b *cold drinks and from exertion.*

**Tart. em.** Cough preceded by crying, or occur after eating or drinking, or when getting warm in bed * Rattling cough, as if the bronchial tubes were ful of mucus, but none is expectorated. * Nausea an vomiting of large quantities of mucus, with cold swea on the forehead. Drowsiness.

**Verat. alb.** Spasmodic cough, with blue face an suffocation. * After every coughing spell the chil falls over exhausted, with cold sweat upon the fore head. * Vomiting of tough, thin mucus, and involun tary discharge of urine. Attacks occur on entering warm room, or from drinking cold water.

---

## PLEURISY.

**Therapeutics.** Special indications.

**Acon.** Chill and synochal fever; full boundin pulse, dry, hot skin, agonized tossing about, violen thirst, red face, shortness of breath, and great nervous excitability. * Piercing and stitching pains in the chest, hindering respiration, with dry cough. Inability to lie on the right side. General suspension of the secretory functions.

**Arnica.** After mechanical injuries. Sensation as if the ribs were bruised. Stitching pains in the left side of the chest, with a short, dry cough. * Sore feeling through the whole system as if from a bruise. * Constantly changing about on account of the bed feeling so hard.

**Bry.** Cheeks flushed and hot. Position upon the affected side with respiration greatly oppressed. * Stitching pain in the affected part, aggravated by inspiration or the least motion. * Headache as if it would split open. * Cannot sit up on account of nausea and faintness. Thirst for large quantities of water at long intervals. * Constipation of hard, dry stools as if burnt. Exceedingly irritable, everything makes him angry.

**Kali c.** When the violent, stitching pain does not yield to *Bryonia.* Darting, stitching, shooting or cutting pains, especially in the right side of the chest. Violent palpitation of the heart. Dry cough, worse about 3 A. M.

**Merc.** Soreness and burning in the chest. Stitching pain in the right side of the chest, through from the shoulder-blade. Cough, aggravated at night and when lying on the left side. Moist tongue, with great thirst. * Much perspiration which does not relieve. * Symptoms all worse at night.

**Phos.** Short, difficult respiration. Lancinating pains, mostly on the left side. Sharp pains when pressing upon the intercostal space. Sense of *tightness* across the chest, with a dry shaking cough. * Sensation of weakness and emptiness in the abdomen. Sharp cutting pains in the bowels, sometimes with vomiting. * Long, narrow, hard stools, very difficult to expel.

**Rhus t.** If the disease has arisen from metastasis of rheumatism, or from exposure to wet, straining, lifting, &c. In cases also where the febrile symptoms have subsided, and there yet remain wandering pains in the chest, shortness of breath, and general debility. * The pains are worse during rest; he has to move continually to get a little relief.

**Squill.** Dyspnœa, with stitching pains in the left side when breathing or coughing. Short rattling cough, disturbing sleep. Inability to lie on the left side. Twitching of the lips, which are covered with thick yellow crusts, more on the left side. Aggravation in the morning.

**Sulph.** Where the disease is complicated with pneumonia, or does not yield to well chosen remedies. There is still some soreness remaining, felt particularly when moving. Short dry cough, with stitches in the chest, extending through to the left shoulder-blade, worse from the least motion. * Frequent weak faint spells, and flashes of heat. * Constant heat on top of the head.

**Tart. em.** Respiration short and difficult. Burning, dry hot skin, or cold, and covered with perspiration. * Sensation as if the inside of the chest were lined with velvet. * Loose cough, as if much phlegm would be expectorated, but nothing comes up. Vertigo with drowsiness. Threatened paralysis of the lungs.

---

## PNEUMONIA.

**Therapeutics.** Special indications.

**Acon.** High fever, with full, bounding pulse, violent thirst, and shortness of breath. * Great fear and anxiety of mind, with nervous excitability. So giddy, cannot sit up in bed. * Fear of death; he predicts the day he will die. Lancinating pain in the chest, with difficulty of breathing.

**Ars.** Great anxiety and restlessness, with much tossing about. * Rapid prostration of strength, with clammy perspiration on the skin. * Urgent thirst, drinking little and often. Burning pain and heat in the chest. Coldness of the extremities. *Great fear of death.* Worse at night, particularly after midnight. In advanced stages.

**Bell.** Congestion towards the brain, with flushed face and throbbing of the carotids. Violent delirium, with a wild look and desire to escape, strike, bite, or quarrel. Oppression and shortness of breath, with pain in the lower and middle portion of the chest. Expectoration bloody, scant and difficult. Dry, cracked tongue and lips, with great thirst. * Starting and jumping during sleep, with moaning. * Sleepiness but cannot sleep. Aggravation at 3 P. M.

**Bry.** Fever moderate. * Cough, with expectoration of tenacious mucus of a *reddish or rusty color.* Great difficulty of breathing, and acute shooting or *stitching pains* in the side or chest. * The pain is aggravated by breathing or the least motion. * Wants to lie perfectly quiet. Cannot sit up on account of nausea and faintness. * Constipation of hard, dry stools, as if burnt. Exceedingly irritable, everything makes him angry. Delirious talking, with desire to escape.

**Carb. v.** In advanced stages, when there is great prostration of the vital forces. * Sensation of great weakness and fatigue in the chest. Cough by spells, with brownish expectoration. Great paleness of the face and coldness of the extremities. Pulse extremely weak. * Craves cold air, and wants to be fanned all the time. Great foulness of all the secretions.

**Lyc.** Predisposed to tuberculous disease. Circumscribed redness of the cheeks. Copious expectoration mixed with pus. * Fan-like motion of the alæ nasi. Great fear of being left alone. * Red, sand-like sediment in the urine. Aggravation from 4 to 8 P. M.

**Merc.** Bilious pneumonia. Oppressed breathing, with stitches in the right chest through from the shoulder-blade. Cough at first dry, afterwards attended with bloody expectoration. * Great tenderness over region of the stomach and liver. * Profuse sweat, affording no relief. Green, slimy stools, *with tenesmus.*

**Nitrum.** Great dyspnœa, must lie with the head

high. Cough, with cutting, stitching pains in the chest, and bloody expectoration. Stitches in the chest when taking a full breath. * Feeling of great heaviness in the chest, as if a load were pressing the thorax together.

**Phos.** In violent cases. The stitching pains are excited or aggravated by coughing or breathing. * Tightness across the chest, with a dry cough and *rust-colored* sputa. * A large portion of the lung is involved, and there is great dyspnœa. * Sensation of weakness and emptiness in the abdomen. *Long, narrow*, hard stools, very difficult to expel. Tall, slender persons, and others who have a weak conformation of the chest. Very sleepy all the time.

**Rhus t.** The disease threatens to assume a typhoid character. The patient lies in a state of half stupefaction, at times delirious. * Terrible cough, which seems as if it would tear something out of the chest. Expectoration, color of brickdust or bloody. * The pains are aggravated by rest, hence the patient continually moves about to get relief. Very restless at night, particularly in the latter part.

**Sang.** In advanced stages. Great difficulty of breathing. Position upon the back with the head well elevated. Stitching, burning pains in the chest. * Cough, with tough, rust-colored expectoration. Circumscribed redness of the cheeks, particularly in the afternoon.

**Sulph.** In protracted cases, occurring in psoric or scrofulous subjects. The disease threatens to terminate in phthisis. * Much rattling of phlegm in the chest. * Frequent weak, faint spells, and flashes of heat. Cough on deep inspiration, with cutting pain in left chest. Feels suffocated, wants the doors and windows open. * Constant heat on top of the head.

**Tart. em.** Short, difficult, and oppressed breathing. * Loose cough, as if much phlegm would be expectorated, but nothing comes up. Great dyspnœa and fits of suffocation. * Impending paralysis of the lungs. * The inside of the chest feels as if lined with velvet. Bilious pneumonia. Nausea and straining to vomit.

**Verat. v.** In the beginning, when congestion and

inflammation have fairly set in. High fever, with strong, quick pulse. Nausea and vomiting of a glairy mucus. * Sinking, faint feeling in the pit of the stomach. Constant burning distress in the cardiac region. Regularly intermitting pulse.

---

## POISONING.

When poison has been taken into the stomach, the main object should be:

1st. To expel it as quickly as possible by inducing the patient to vomit.

2d. To neutralize its effects by appropriate antidotes.

To excite vomiting, administer copious draughts of tepid water, and tickle the fauces with a feather or something similar. Placing a little salt, snuff, or mustard upon the tongue is very efficient. If these fail, give injections of tobacco-smoke. When emetics are used, *sulphate of zinc* is the most efficient. Twenty-four grains may be given in a little water, and repeated if necessary.

**Poisoning by Acids.** Give: 1, warm soap-suds; 2, magnesia in water; 3, powdered chalk, mixed in warm water; 4, wood-ashes, soda, potash, gruel, linseed-tea, or rice-water.

**Poisoning by Alkalies.** No vomiting. Give: 1, dilute vinegar; 2, lemonade; 3, sour milk; 4, mucilaginous drinks; 5, sweet oil.

**Poisoning by Antimony.** Give a strong decoction of gall-nuts, oak-bark, strong black tea, strong coffee, and mucilaginous drinks.

**Poisoning by Arsenic.** Induce vomiting by tepid water, tickling the throat, placing snuff, salt, or mustard upon the tongue, or use the stomach-pump. The proper antidote is *peroxide of iron*, a spoonful to an adult. If this is not at hand, give *iron-rust* stirred in sugar-water; flaxseed tea, flour and water, white of eggs and water, soap-suds, or calcined magnesia in water. After the alarming symptoms have passed, give *Ipecac.* If the patient is very uneasy at night and irritable, give *China.* If he is worse in the morning, has slimy diarrhœa, or constipation, give *Nux v.* If nausea and vomiting, with heat or chilliness over the whole body and great debility, give *Verat. alb.*

**Poisoning by Cantharides.** Give white of eggs and slimy substances, as gruel, linseed-tea, &c. Afterwards smell *Camph.*, or take it internally.

**Poisoning by Copper.** Excite vomiting. Give white of eggs, sugar-water, milk, and mucilaginous drinks.

**Poisoning by Corrosive Sublimate.** Excite vomiting immediately. Give *white of eggs*, beaten up in water, in large quantities. Next in importance is *sugar-water*, starch boiled in water, flour-paste, and milk in large quantities.

**Poisoning by Iodine.** Excite vomiting by a weak solution of soda. Give starch stirred in water, thin starch-paste, flour-paste, linseed-tea, &c.

**Poisoning by Gases.** Charcoal Gas.—If a person has become insensible from inhaling this gas, expose him at once to the fresh air, bathe the face and breast with *vinegar*, and give him strong coffee. After he has somewhat recovered, dispense with the vinegar, and give *Opium.* If this does not suffice, give *Bell.* or *Nux v.* Dr. Hall's method of inducing artificial respiration, as explained on page 16, should be resorted to, if necessary.

**Poisoning by Lead.** For poisoning by sugar of lead and other preparations, *excite vomiting.* Give: 1, Epsom Salts; 2, Glauber Salts; 3, white of eggs; 4, soap-suds; 5, milk.

**Poisoning by Nitrate of Silver.** Give: 1, Common salt dissolved in water, in large quantities; 2, mucilaginous drinks.

**Poisoning by Opium.** Excite vomiting, or use the stomach-pump. The best antidote is *strong coffee*; until that can be had, give vinegar and water. Keep the patient roused by beating him on the back and dragging him about the room. Artificial respiration should be induced, as explained under "Apparent Death from Drowning," page 16.

**Poisoning by Phosphorus.** Excite vomiting. Give: 1, Magnesia stirred in water; 2, mucilaginous drinks in large quantities. Chlorine water and magnesia, eight parts of the former to one of the latter, a spoonful taken every five or ten minutes.

**Poisoning by Prussic Acid.** Give Spirits of Hartshorn to smell, and a weak solution internally. Pour cold water down the spine from a height, give strong coffee to drink, and use the same as an injection.

**Poisoning by Stramonium.** Give: 1, Coffee; 2, vinegar; 3, lemonade in large quantities.

**Poisoning by Strychnine.** Evacuate the stomach as quickly as possible by tepid water and tickling the throat; give an emetic of *sulphate of zinc*, or use the stomach-pump. The antidotes recommended are, *Iodine* (30 drops in water), *Camphor* (5 grains dissolved in mucilage). These, it is said, stop the tetanic spasms, and give time for the action of the stomach-pump, or emetic.

---

## PUERPERAL CONVULSIONS.

**Therapeutics.** Special indications.

**Acon.** In the incipiency, when an attack is apprehended. Flushed face, dry, hot skin, thirst, and great restlessness. * Great fear and anxiety of mind, thinks she will die, although there is no occasion of alarm. * She dreads too much activity about her. Vertigo on rising up in bed.

**Argen. n.** The patient has a presentiment of the approaching spasm. Tremor of the limbs, and faintish, weak feeling. * Sensation as if the body, and especially the face and head, expanded. She feels as if the bones of the skull separated with increase of temperature. * Continually in motion between the spasms.

**Bell.** Red, bloated face, with distorted eyes and dilated pupils. * She seems to be in a half-conscious state, with disposition to strike, bite, or injure those about her. Convulsive jerking of the limbs and muscles of the face. Foam at the mouth, and involuntary escape of fæces and urine. With every pain a spasm comes on, and during the interval more or less tossing about. * Sensation as if she were falling down through the bed. Paralysis of the right side of the tongue; difficult deglutition.

**Cham.** Great irritability of temper, she can hardly give one a civil answer. * Red, bloated face, or one cheek red and the other pale. Becomes furious about the pains, which are spasmodic and distressing. * Twitching of the muscles of the face and eyelids. Great impatience, restlessness, and nervous excitability. Starting during sleep, with dry, hot skin.

**Cicu.** Violent contortions of the upper part of the body and limbs. Convulsive tossing of the extremities from one side to another. * Bluish face with interrupted breathing and foam at the mouth. * After the convulsion she lies motionless, with rigidity of the jaws, and as if dead.

**Cup.** The spasm sets in with sudden convulsive jerking of the limbs. The arms are drawn in towards the body, and the fingers tightly clenched. Eyes spasmodically closed, and the mouth distorted. * Rigidity of the trunk and lower extremities, with closed jaws. * Vomiting and retching, with horrible colic and cramps in the legs.

**Hyos.** The spasms commence with twitching of the muscles of the face, and spasmodic motions of the eyelids. * Twitching and jerking of all the muscles in the body. * Clenching of the thumbs in the palms of the hands. Complete loss of consciousness, throwing off the bed-clothing, and endeavoring to escape. Oppression of the chest, *with stertorous breathing.* Involuntary discharge of fæces and urine.

**Ign.** * Sudden starting from sleep, with screams, and trembling of the whole body. Twitching of the muscles of the face and corners of the mouth. Convulsive movements of single muscles, or only portions of the body at a time. * Deep sighing and sobbing, with a strange compressed feeling in the brain.

**Opi.** Particularly if caused by fright. Convulsive

trembling of the whole body, with distortion of the muscles. * The spasm is followed by sopor and stertorous respiration. * Stupefaction of the senses, and complete loss of consciousness. Bluish, bloated face, with swollen lips. Pupils dilated and insensible to light. Incoherent and wandering talk. Hot perspiration about the head and face.

**Stram.** * The patient awakens with a shrinking look, as if afraid of the first object seen. The spasm mostly commences with convulsive motions of the extremities, especially the upper. Spasmodic drawing in the head and eyes, with grinding of the teeth. * Loquacious delirium, with stammering speech. She makes ridiculous gestures and strange faces; laughs, sings, and sighs. * The light of brilliant objects, and contact, renew the spasms.

---

## RHEUMATISM.

**Therapeutics.** Special indications.

**Acon.** Synochal fever, with dry hot skin and great thirst. Red shining swelling of the affected part, *very sensitive to contact and motion.* Stitching pains in the chest, hindering free respiration. * Great fear and anxiety of mind, with great nervous excitability. Retention of urine, and stitches in the kidneys.

**Amm. phos.** Especially where the joints of the fingers and hands are involved. Loss of appetite, with emaciation. Sleeplessness and nervous irritability. Mostly the *right side* of the body. Evening fever.

**Arn.** Hard, red, and shining swelling of the affected parts. * Pains as if sprained or bruised, with a feeling of lameness in the affected limb * Sensation as if the diseased part were resting upon something hard. * Great fear of being struck by persons coming near him.

**Ars.** Burning, stinging, tearing pain, with pale swelling of the parts. * Pain relieved by the application of warmth, and aggravated by cold. Profuse sweat, which relieves the pain, but leaves the patient very weak. Frequent chills, alternating with heat. Constantly moving the affected limbs. * Extreme thirst, drinking little and often.

**Bell.** Red shining swelling of the joints, with pressing, cutting, tearing pain, deep in the bones. * Frequent darting pains from the joint along the limb. * Pains which come on suddenly, and leave as suddenly. Fever, with dry hot skin, thirst, and throbbing headache. Visible pulsations of the carotids. Drowsy, sleepy condition, with starting and jumping during sleep. Aggravation at 3 P. M., and from the least motion or touch.

**Bry.** Stiffness, with swelling and a faintish redness of the inflamed part. * Stitching, tearing pains, worse from the slightest motion. * The patient wants to remain perfectly still. Dry hot skin, or else perspiration of an acrid character. Bitter taste, dry mouth and lips, with great thirst for large quantities of water. * Hard, dry stools, as if burnt. Exceedingly *irritable.* Metastasis to the heart.

**Cactus.** The disease is principally confined to the heart and diaphragm. * Feeling as if an iron band was around the heart, preventing its normal action. Palpitation of the heart, worse when lying on the left side.

**Caulophyl.** * Rheumatism of the wrists and finger-joints, with much swelling. When the disease shifts from the extremities to the back and nape of the neck, with rigidity of the muscles. Oppression of the chest, and high fever.

**Caust.** Stiffness and swelling of the joints, with tearing pains. * Great weakness and lameness of the lower limbs, and trembling of the hands. Pains worse towards evening, and from exposure to cold; better from the external application of heat. Scrofulous persons, with yellow complexion.

**Cham.** Drawing or tearing pains, with a sensation of numbness or lameness in the affected parts. The pains are continuous, and get worse at night, with much tossing about. * Becomes almost furious about the pains, can hardly endure them. * Great irritability, can hardly answer a civil question. Hot perspiration, especially about the head. * Redness of one cheek, and paleness of the other.

**Chelidonium.** * Rheumatic swelling, with a *stone-like hardness* of the affected parts. Constant pain under the lower inner angle of the right shoulder-blade. * Stools like sheep's-dung.

**China.** Violent, tearing, sticking, drawing pains, increased by pressure or motion. Bruised pains in the small of the back, with occasional painful jerks in the region of the os sacrum. *Debilitating morning and night sweats.* * Weakly persons, who have lost much blood.

**Cimicifu.** Articular rheumatism of the lower extremities, with much swelling and heat of the affected parts. Pain worse from motion, extorting screams. Delicate hysterical females who suffer from uterine diseases.

**Colch.** Moderate swelling, with pale redness of the affected parts. Pains burning, tearing, or jerking, and frequently shifting about. * Chilliness even near the hot stove, intermingled with flashes of heat. Metastasis to the heart, with stitches and tearing in the chest and region of the heart, during an inspiration. Strong and fluttering beating of the heart. Profuse *sour-smelling sweats.* * Urine dark and scanty, depositing a whitish sediment.

**Dulc.** If caused by cold or dampness. The parts feel as if bruised or beaten. The pains are mostly in the back, joints of the arms, and legs. When the disease sets in after acute cutaneous eruptions. * Aggravation after every cold change in the weather.

**Ferr.** Little or no swelling, but a constant drawing, tearing pain, especially in the deltoid muscle. Pain worse in bed; has to get up and walk slowly about. * Least emotion or exertion produces a red flushed face. Palpitation of the heart, and dyspnœa.

**Hama.** Pains unbearable, with great sensitiveness to touch, and fear of exciting new pain on moving. * Great soreness of the affected parts. Articular rheumatism, with swollen and painful joints.

**Kreos.** Pain in the joints, especially in the hip and knee-joints, with a feeling of numbness or loss of sensation, as though the whole limb were going to sleep. * Wretched livid complexion.

**Lach.** Swelling of the index-finger and wrist-joint. Stinging, tearing pains in the knees, with a sense of swelling. Left side generally most affected. No relief from profuse sweating. * Patient worse after sleeping.

**Ledum.** Rheumatic pains in the lower extremities, especially in the hip and knee-joints, and when it commences from below and goes upwards. * Great want of vital heat. Pains grow worse in the evening in bed, and last till midnight.

**Lyc.** Drawing and tearing pains, worse at night and during rest. Painful rigidity of the muscles and joints, with sensation of numbness in the affected part. The disease is mostly on the right side, with or without swelling. Chronic forms, especially of old people. * Urine dark and turbid, or with *sediment of red sand.* * Constant sensation of satiety, feels so full can eat nothing. Constipation, much sour belching.

**Merc.** Shooting, tearing, or burning pains, worse at night, from the warmth of the bed or exposure to damp or cold air. Puffy swelling of the affected parts, of a pale or slight pinkish color. Green, slimy diarrhœa, with griping and tenesmus. * Much perspiration, affording no relief.

**Nux v.** Rheumatism, especially of the back, loins, chest, or joints, with pale, tensive swelling. Tensive, jerking, or pulling pains aggravated by contact or motion. Numbness or lameness of the affected parts, with twitching in the muscles. Aversion to the open air, and great sensitiveness to cold. Heat mixed with chilliness, especially when moving. * Perspiration relieves the pain. Dyspeptic symptoms. * Habitual constipation. Persons of intemperate habits. Irritable mood.

**Phos.** Tearing, drawing, and tensive pains setting in when taking the least cold. Sense of lameness and weakness in the lower limbs. * Sensation of weakness and emptiness in the abdomen. Belching up large quantities of wind after eating. * Long, narrow, hard stools, very difficult to expel.

**Puls.** Not much swelling or redness of the affected

parts. Pains drawing, tearing, and jerking, worse at night or in the evening in bed. * Pains which shift rapidly from one part to another. Sensation of weight in the disordered structure. * Chilliness even in a warm room. * Craves cold, fresh air; feels worse in a warm temperature. * Persons of a mild, tearful disposition. * Bad taste in the mouth in the morning.

**Rhod**. Drawing, tearing pains in the joints and limbs. Pains worse during rest, and in rough stormy weather. Swelling and redness of single joints. *Rheumatism of the knee.*

**Rhus t.** Swelling and redness of the affected part. Pains drawing, tearing, burning, or as if sprained, with sensation of lameness and creeping in the parts. * Pains worse during rest and when first commencing to move. * Better from continued motion and external warm applications.

**Spig**. Rheumatic pericarditis. Dull stitches in the region where the beats of the heart are felt. Violent palpitation of the heart, with great anxiety. Dyspnœa, he can lie only on the right side, with the trunk raised. * The least motion produces great suffocation.

**Sulph**. Chronic form, and for the secondary effects of acute rheumatism. Tearing, stitching, or dull aching pains. * Constant heat in top of the head. * Frequent weak, faint spells.

**Thuya**. Tearing and beating pains, as if from subcutaneous ulceration. Feeling of coldness and numbness in the affected parts. Rheumatism in syphilitic subjects. Symptoms worse in a warm temperature.

**Verat. a**. Pains as if bruised, worse from the heat of the bed; better from rising and walking about. * Electric jerks in the affected limbs. Painful heaviness in the knees and lower legs.

**Verat. v**. Rheumatism, especially of the left shoulder, hip, and knee. Advised in endocarditis and pericarditis.

## SCARLATINA.

**Therapeutics.** Special indications.

**Acon.** Mostly in the commencement, before the eruption makes its appearance. Dry hot skin, with full frequent pulse, agonized tossing about, violent thirst, and hurried breathing. * Great fear and anxiety of mind, with great nervous excitability. Pain in the stomach, with nausea and vomiting.

**Amm. c.** Hard swelling of the parotid and lymphatic glands of the neck. The rash continues out longer than the usual period. * There is a tendency to gangrenous ulceration. Nose obstructed.

**Apis m.** Fever of a typhoid character. Tongue of a deep-red color, and covered with blisters. * Nose discharges a thick, white, fetid, or bloody mucus. Tonsils swollen and hard, with difficult deglutition. *Ulcerated throat.* Abdomen sore to the touch. Dropsical symptoms during desquamation. Child lies in a stupor.

**Ars.** When the eruption delays or grows suddenly pale, *with rapid prostration.* Putrid sore-throat. * Great anguish, extreme restlessness, and fear of death. * Intense thirst, drinking little and often. Internal heat, with external coldness. Fetid diarrhœa.

**Arum tri.** Corners of the mouth and lips sore and cracked. Redness of the tongue, with elevated papillæ. Throat extremely sore and putrid. Submaxillary glands swollen. * Nose stopped up, or discharging a burning ichorous fluid, excoriating the nostrils and upper lip. Eruption all over the body, with much itching and restlessness. * Scarlatina maligna.

**Baryta c.** Parotid and submaxillary glands swollen, with much saliva, or else dryness of the throat. Tonsils swollen, and of a pale-red color, with pressing, stinging pain on swallowing. Breath putrid. * Scrofulous children that grow but little.

**Bell.** * The eruption is perfectly smooth and of a scarlet color. Skin so hot that it imparts a burning sensation to the hand. Tongue white, with red edges and prominent papillæ. Fauces inflamed and of a *deep red color.* Throat swollen outside, and tender to touch. * Congestion to the brain, with delirium, and throbbing of the carotids. * Starting and jumping while sleeping. Springs suddenly up in bed, and attempts to escape.

**Bry.** The eruption does not come out fully, or suddenly disappears. Congestion to the chest with difficult, anxious respiration. Sensation of weight upon the chest, with troublesome cough. Headache as if it would split open, worse by motion. Lips parched, dry, and cracked. * Patient wants to lie perfectly still.

**Calc. c.** In protracted cases, where the glands of the neck are swollen and hard. Throat greatly inflamed, with aphthæ on the tonsils and roof of the mouth. Does not convalesce after the regular recession of the eruption. Face pale and bloated, showing no signs of rash. * Scrofulous persons, and children with large open fontanels.

**Camph.** In desperate cases. Extremities cold and purple. Rattling in the throat, and hot breath. Hot perspiration on the forehead; the child refuses to be covered. Sudden retrocession of the eruption.

**Carb. v.** Usually in the last stage. * Putrid sore throat, with sloughing of the fauces. Rattling in the throat. Great prostration of strength, with cold breath, and coldness of the extremities. *Craves cold air.*

**Cup. acet.** * When *metastasis to the brain is apprehended,* or the eruption suddenly disappears, followed by convulsions, vomiting, and gagging. Rolling of the eyes, distortions of the face and all the flexor muscles. Great restlessness and tossing about. Sopor and delirium.

**Ipec.** Slight fever through the day, increased in the evening. * Constant nausea and vomiting of green, bilious, or slimy matter. Great uneasiness in the stomach and epigastrium. Violent itching of the skin. Sleeplessness, with sadness and despondency.

**Kali c.** Swelling of the right parotid gland. Great dryness, stinging, and itching of the skin. Stinging pain in the throat when swallowing. * Puffiness under the eyebrows like little bags. Always worse about three o'clock in the morning.

**Lach.** Scarlatina maligna, with external swelling of the neck and glands. Diphtheric inflammation of the throat, with great difficulty in swallowing. * External throat very painful to touch. Ulcers on the tongue. * Aggravation after sleeping.

**Lyc.** Inflammation of the throat of a brownish-red color, with stitches on swallowing. * Ulceration of the tonsils, beginning on the right and spreading to the left. Obstruction of the nose. Rattling in the throat, and hawking up of bloody mucus. Dryness of the mouth and tongue, without thirst. * Red sediment like sand in the urine.

**Merc.** Ulcers from the mouth, throat, and upon the tonsils, covered with ash-colored sloughs. Deglutition very difficult, attended with a stinging pain. Fluids escape through the mouth and nose when he attempts to swallow. Very fetid breath. * Profuse secretion of saliva, often offensive. Acrid discharge from the nose.

**Mur. ac.** Malignant cases, where the tonsils and throat are swollen, inflamed, and covered with dark-colored ulcers. Great tendency for the sloughs to extend and run together. Dark-redness of the face, and purplish color of the skin. Discharge of thin, acrid pus from the nose, excoriating the parts around. * Sliding down in the bed.

**Nitr. ac.** Putrid sore throat extending up into the nose. Profuse discharge of thin, purulent matter from the nostrils. *Putrid-smelling breath; mouth full of fetid ulcers.* Swelling of the parotid and submaxillary glands. Ulceration of the corners of the mouth and lips. After the abuse of mercury.

**Opi.** * Extreme drowsiness, stertorous breathing and vomiting. Delirious talking, with eyes wide open, face red and puffed up. * Impending paralysis of the brain.

**Rhus t.** The rash is dark-colored and *itches violently.* Tongue red and smooth, with drowsiness and delirium. Much fever and restlessness, particularly after midnight. Swelling of the glands in the throat, and an ichorous or yellow, thick discharge from the nose. * Constantly changing position to obtain relief.

**Zinc**. * Threatening paralysis of the brain. The child lies in a state of unconsciousness. Jerking of the whole body, or twitching of single limbs. Grating of the teeth, and shrill, frightful screams during sleep. Small, frequent pulse, and fixed, stupid expression of the eyes. Icy coldness of the skin from sunken vitality.

For the troublesome sequelæ, which often follow scarlet fever, the following remedies will be found especially appropriate: **Apis m., Ars., Aurum m., Baryta c., Bell., Dig., Hell., Kali c., Lyc., Phos., Puls., Rhus t., Sulph.,** and **Verat. a.**

As a disinfectant in this and other diseases of like character, *Chlorate of Potassa* is of great value. Dissolve half an ounce of the salt in three pints of water; saturate clothes in the solution and hang them about the room. *Carbolic acid* is likewise a deodorizer of much value, and extensively used at the present time.

---

## SMALL-POX.

**Therapeutics.** Special indications.

**Acon.** At the commencement, during the febrile stage, especially if there be congestion to the head or lungs. Headache, bleeding at the nose, and injected eyes. Fulness in the chest, with increased action of the heart. Pain in the back, and aching in the limbs.

**Apis m.** If there is an erysipelatous redness and swelling, with stinging burning pains. * Stinging and burning pains in the throat. * Sensation in the abdomen as if something tight would break.

**Ars.** The eruption is very dark, and the skin turns blue or livid. Great sinking of strength, small frequent pulse, and restlessness. * Extreme thirst, drinking little and often. * Great anguish and fear of death.

**Bell.** Congestion to the head, with throbbing or stitching pain in the forehead. High fever and sore throat. * Starting and jumping during sleep. Restless tossing about, cannot get to sleep. * Pain in the back as if it would break.

**Camph.** Sudden desiccation of the pustules and disappearance of the swelling of the face. * Extreme prostration and sinking of the vital forces. * Great coldness of the skin, but cannot bear to be covered.

**Hydras.** Great redness, swelling, and itching of the skin, with very sore throat. It is said to prevent pitting to a great extent.

**Merc.** During the suppurative stage. *Ulcerated throat, with profuse flow of saliva.* Diarrhœa, with green or bloody mucous stools, with tenesmus. * Perspiration without relief.

**Opi.** If the brain becomes oppressed, and there is great drowsiness, with stertorous breathing. * Complete loss of consciousness. Dilated pupils.

**Rhus t.** The disease has assumed a typhoid character. Tongue dry and cracked, corners of the mouth sore and ulcerated. Sordes on the lips and teeth, mind wandering. Great debility and restlessness. * Worse after midnight.

**Sulph.** In the early stage, and about the period of desiccation; also as an intercurrent remedy when others seem to fail.

**Tart. em.** This remedy has been found to greatly ameliorate the disease. It reduces the fever, and the pustules run their course, leaving scarcely a mark behind. Especially suited where there is much irritation of the respiratory organs.

**Vaccinin** and **Variolin** have been highly extolled as remedies in this disease. It is said, by those who have used them extensively, that all stages of the malady are shortened, and the disease rendered mild and harmless. * They promote suppuration and exsiccation, and prevent all scars.

## SPASMS.

**Therapeutics.** Special indications.

**Acon.** High fever, with dry, hot skin, anxiety, and restlessness. During dentition. If caused from the irritation of ascarides. Grinding of the teeth and convulsive hiccough.

**Arn.** Where the spasms arise in consequence of some mechanical injury, from concussion of the brain, a fall or blow.

**Ars.** Spasms preceded by great restlessness, and burning heat over the whole body. *Extreme thirst, drinking little and often. Patient lies motionless as if dead; finally, the mouth is drawn first to one side and then to the other; a violent jerk appears to pass through the whole body, and consciousness gradually returns.

**Bell.** Heat of the head, with flushed face, red eyes, and dilated pupils. *Starting and jumping during sleep. Drowsiness with inability to sleep. Convulsive motion of the mouth, facial muscles, and eyes. Foam at the mouth, and grating of the teeth. *Drowsiness after the spasm. *Precocious* children.

**Caust.** Convulsive motions of the extremities, grinding of the teeth, laughing or weeping. Feverish heat of the body, with coldness of the hands and feet. Cold water brings on the spasms again.

**Cham.** Stretching of the limbs, with convulsions of the extremities, eyes, eyelids, and tongue. Jerking and twitching during sleep. *Redness of the face, or one cheek red and the other pale. *The child is very cross and fretful, must be carried all the time to be quieted. Hot sweat on the forehead and hairy scalp. Constant moaning and craving for drink.

**Cicu.** Spasmodic rigidity of the body, with the head bent either backward or forward. *Without any premonitory signs the child becomes suddenly stiff, with fixed eyes. After the spasm there is much prostration. If the convulsions are caused by worms.

**Cina.** Spasms of the chest, followed by rigidity of the limbs or the whole body. Especially suited to children troubled with worms. * Constantly picking and boring at the nose. Frequent swallowing, as if something were in the throat. Dry hacking cough. Urine turns milky after standing.

**Cupr.** Shrill cries during the attack. Drowsy and stupid during the intervals, with nausea and vomiting of phlegm. * After the convulsion, the child screams, turns and twists in all directions. If caused from retrocession of scarlatina eruption.

**Gels.** Spasms during dentition, with sudden loud outcries. Nervous, excitable persons who are very sensitive.

**Hyos.** Convulsions with twitching and jerking of all the muscles, especially those about the face and eyes. * Convulsive trembling and foam at the mouth. After sudden fright. * Cough, worse when lying down, relieved by sitting up.

**Ign.** Sudden starting from a light sleep, with loud screaming and trembling all over. * Single parts seem to be convulsed, or single muscles here and there. * The spasms return every day or every other day about the same hour.

**Ipec.** * Much nausea and vomiting accompanies the spasms. Especially if caused by eating indigestible food, or when during an exanthematic fever the eruption suddenly strikes in. *Green* diarrhœic stools.

**Opi.** Trembling over the whole body, and tossing about of the limbs. * Loud screaming before or during the spasm. The child lies unconscious as if stunned, with heavy difficult breathing. * Convulsions caused from fright.

**Secale.** Twitching of single muscles. Twisting of the head to and fro. Contortions of the hands and feet. Labored and anxious respiration. * Thin, scrawny children, with shrivelled skin.

**Sili.** * Spasms which return at the change of the moon. Much perspiration about the head. * Constipation, the stool recedes after having been partially expelled.

**Stram.** Convulsions from fright, with tossing of the limbs, and involuntary evacuations of fæces and urine. * Awakens with a shrinking look, as if afraid of the first object seen. If caused by suppressed eruptions, or the eruption does not come out sufficiently.

**Sulph.** After suppressed eruptions. * Comes out of the spasm very happy, and at the termination of the paroxysm passes much colorless urine. * Morning diarrhœa. Spasms during the eruptive stage of scarlatina.

**Zinc.** * The child cries out during sleep, and seems frightened when getting awake, rolls its head from side to side. Twitching and jerking of different muscles, more on the right side than on the left. Cross and irritable. Frequent passages of urine.

---

## SUNSTROKE.

**Therapeutics.** Special indications.

**Acon.** If the head has been exposed to the direct rays of the sun. Violent thirst, red face, shortness of breath, and great nervous excitability.

**Bell.** Severe headache and fulness, as if the head would split, worse when stooping. Feeling in the forehead as if the brain would be pressed out. * Vertigo when stooping or rising from a sitting posture.

**Bry.** Headache as if it would split open, aggravated by the least motion. Very peevish in the morning, is more passionate and cross than plaintive. * Cannot sit up from nausea and faintness. * Dry, hard stools as if burnt. Head feels *too full.*

**Carb. v.** Headache, heaviness, throbbing, and pressure over the eyes. Pains in the eyes, aggravated by looking fixedly at any object.

**Glonoine.** This remedy has been used with great benefit in sunstroke. It is indicated by: Intense congestion of blood to the head. Feeling as if the temples and top of the head would burst open. * Violent, throbbing headache, with increased action of the heart. Fulness and pressure in forepart and top of the head, with confusion of the senses. * Sensation of balancing, requiring a constant effort to keep the head erect.

Undulating sensation, increased by every turn of the head. Sick, faint, death-like sinking at the epigastrium, with nausea.

---

## TONSILLITIS.

**Therapeutics.** Special indications.

**Acon.** Tonsils swollen, inflamed, and of a dark-red color, accompanied by a high grade of fever. Pain and great difficulty in swallowing or in speaking. Burning, pricking, or contracting sensation in the throat. * Great restlessness and nervous excitability.

**Amm. m.** Swelling and inflammation of both tonsils. The patient can neither swallow, talk, nor open his mouth. When cold is the exciting cause. * Tendency to gangrenous ulceration.

**Apis m.** Red and highly inflamed tonsils, with dryness in the mouth and throat. * Burning, stinging pain in the throat when swallowing. Can bear nothing to touch his neck. Aggravation from heat, better from cold.

**Baryta c.** Raw, scraping, or shooting pain when swallowing. Sensation as if a plug were in the throat. * The tonsils incline to suppurate. * Chronic induration of the tonsils.

**Bell.** Tonsils swollen, inflamed, and of a dark-red color; the swelling perceptible on the outside. Burning and shooting pains in the throat when swallowing. * The throat feels as if a plug were in it. * Drinking produces spasms in the throat, the fluids returning through the nose. Constant inclination to swallow or hawk up something. Especially if on the right side.

**Hepar s.** Where there is a frequent recurrence of the disease. Sticking pain, as from a fish-bone in the throat, when swallowing. * Inclination to suppurate. Persons of a scrofulous habit. After the abuse of mercury.

**Lach.** Tonsillitis, especially on the left side. When

swallowing, the pain extends to the ear. Fluids escape through the nose when being swallowed. Sensation of a plug or lump in the throat. Ulcers on the throat. * Cannot bear anything to touch the neck, not even the bed-clothes. * Worse in the afternoon, and after sleep.

**Merc.** Tonsils swollen, inflamed, and dark-red, or become ulcerated. Offensive odor from the mouth. Aphthæ. or thick yellow coating on the tongue. Violent pricking pains when swallowing, extending to the ears or glands of the throat. Gums and back part of the tongue swollen. * Profuse discharge of saliva. * Much perspiration, which does not relieve. Aggravation during the night.

**Nux v.** If derangement of the stomach be the predisposing cause. Sensation as if a plug or lump were in the throat when swallowing. The throat feels raw and excoriated, or as if scraped and rough. * Patient very irritable, and wishes to be alone. Dyspeptics and persons who have been drugged with mixtures. Symptoms worse in the morning.

**Sili.** When the appearance of the throat indicates the *formation of an abscess*, attended with stitches and throbbing pain. Mostly on the left side. Scrofulous persons.

**Sulph.** Where there is a frequent recurrence of the disease. After the abscesses burst, the parts remain sore, and do not heal as they should. Scrofulous persons who are troubled with boils; every little scratch of the skin has a tendency to fester. * Lean persons who walk stooping. * Frequent weak faint spells.

---

## TOOTHACHE.

**Therapeutics.** Special indications.

**Acon.** The patient is almost frantic with the pain, which is indescribable. Stitching or throbbing pains, with congestion of blood to the head, and great restlessness. * Constant fear and anxiety of mind, with great nervous excitability.

**Ant. cr.** Pains in carious teeth, followed by jerking and gnawing, extending up to the head, especially in the evening, in bed. Pains worse after eating, or from cold water: better in the open air. The gums bleed readily, and recede from the teeth.

**Arn.** *Toothache after an operation.* Pain as if the teeth were sprained. *Cheek swollen, red, and hard,* with beating and tingling in the gums. * Sore, bruised feeling all through the patient.

**Ars.** Elongation and painful looseness of the teeth. Drawing, jerking pains in the teeth and gums, extending to the ears, cheeks, and temples. The pains are so great that they drive the patient to despair. *Prostration; restlessness; drinking often and but little.*

**Bell.** Drawing, tearing pains in the teeth, face, and ears, with swelling of the cheek. Ptyalism, or dryness of the throat and mouth, with great thirst. * Pains which come on suddenly, and leave just as suddenly. Face flushed, and eyes red. Pains worse after lying down at night, or in the cold air.

**Bry.** Pains in carious, and still more in sound teeth. *Sensation of elongation* in the teeth, with jerking, drawing pains. Worse at night, or from taking anything warm in the mouth. Mouth unusually dry, with thirst. * Constipation, stools dry and hard, as if burnt. Exceedingly irritable. Wants to be perfectly still.

**Calc. c.** Beating, stitching, boring pains, or soreness of the teeth. * The pains are aggravated by a draught of air, by drinking anything *warm* or *cold,* or by the slightest change.

**Carb. v.** Receding and bleeding gums, with ulcers. The teeth are loose, and sensitive to contact, especially after eating. * The pains come on and are made worse from eating salt things.

**Cham.** After taking cold when in a perspiration. The pains are drawing, jerking, or *beating* and *stitching.* Intolerable pains, especially at night, driving one to despair. Hot swelling of the cheeks, and red swollen gums. * Becomes almost furious about the pains; worse in the open air and at night. * Very impatient, can scarcely give a civil answer.

**China.** The pain comes on periodically, and is throbbing, tearing, jerking, or drawing. Aggravation from the slightest *contact*, from a draught of air, or from smoking; relieved by pressing the teeth firmly together. * Nursing females, and persons debilitated from loss of animal fluids.

**Coff.** Insupportable pains, which drive the patient almost frantic. * The pain is relieved by ice-cold water. * Head feels contracted or too small. * Excessive wakefulness. Loss of taste.

**Dulc.** Toothache from taking cold in damp or wet weather, and if accompanied by diarrhœa. Confusion of the head and profuse salivation. The teeth feel blunt. * Symptoms always worse by a cold change in the weather.

**Hepar.** Painful swelling of the cheeks. Jerking and drawing pains in the teeth, worse when pressing the teeth together, when eating, in a warm room, or *at night.*

**Hyos.** Pains which almost drive the patient mad; it is a tearing or throbbing, extending to the cheeks and along the lower jaw. Swelling of the gums, with a tearing pain and buzzing in the tooth, which appears loose. * Spasmodic twitching of the fingers, hands, arms, and facial muscles. Aggravation in the morning and from cold air.

**Merc.** Tearing pains in several teeth at one time, affecting the whole side of the face. Drawing and stinging pains, which extend to the ear, or jumping pains in the teeth, especially at night. The pains are excited by cool damp air, or by eating anything hot or cold. * The teeth feel sore, loose, and too long. * Perspiration does not relieve. *Much saliva in the mouth.*

**Meze.** Carious teeth are principally affected. The pains are burning, boring, or drawing stitches. * When the pains extend to the bones of the face and temples. Worse by contact, motion, or in the evening, with chilliness.

**Nux v.** Sore pains or jerking, drawing, with

stitches in the teeth and jaw. Pains extending to the head, ears, and malar bones, with painful swelling of the submaxillary glands. Aggravation at night, or early in *the morning*, from mental labor and in a warm room; better in the open air. * He feels cross and irritable. * Persons of sedentary habits, and who live upon exciting or stimulating food.

**Puls.** Suited to persons of a mild, tearful disposition. Toothache, with otalgia and hemicrania. Pains tearing, drawing, stitching, or jerking, as if the nerves were put upon the stretch, and then suddenly let go again. * Better from cold things, and worse from warm. * Chilliness even in a warm room. *Scanty or suppressed menses.*

**Rhus t.** The teeth feel loose and too long. Gums swollen; they burn and itch like an ulcer. Jumping, shooting, or drawing pains, as if the teeth were being torn out. * Aggravated during rest and in damp weather. * Better from the application of external heat.

**Sepia.** Toothache *during pregnancy*. The pains are beating, stitching, and extend to the ears, and along the arm to the fingers, where they terminate in a creeping sensation. *Swelling of the cheeks* and submaxillary glands, with cough. * Sallow complexion, with spots on the face. *Profuse leucorrhœa* having a fetid smell.

**Spig.** Tearing, shooting, or burning pains, with dark redness of the affected side. Flow of water from the eyes and nose. Pains worse from applying cold water or going into the open air. *Palpitation of the heart, chilliness, restlessness.

**Staph.** * Black, carious teeth which incline to crumble. *Pale, white, ulcerated, swollen and painful gums.* Aching, tearing, and drawing pains in carious and in the roots of sound teeth. Worse early in the morning and after drinking anything cold. Cold sweat in the face, and cold hands.

**Sulph.** Jumping pain in hollow teeth, extending to the upper and lower jaw, or to the ears. Looseness, elongation or dulness of the teeth. Aggravation or renewal of the pains in the evening or at night in bed, or from *cold water*. * Burning heat in top of the head, and cold extremities. * Scanty, black menstrual discharges.

---

## TYPHOID FEVER.

**Therapeutics.** Special indications.

**Acon.** Chill and synochal fever, with full, bounding pulse, great heat, dry, burning skin and violent thirst. * Great fear and anxiety of mind, with much nervous excitability. * Headache as if everything would press out of the forehead, with vertigo on rising up. Mostly in the first stage.

**Apis m.** The patient remains in a stupid unconscious state, with muttering delirium. Inability to talk or put out the tongue, which is cracked, ulcerated, or covered with vesicles. Dryness of the mouth and throat, with difficulty of swallowing. * Great soreness in the pit of the stomach and abdomen when touched. Constipation, or frequent, foul, bloody mucus and involuntary stools. White miliary eruption on the chest and abdomen. * Great weakness and sliding down in bed.

**Arn.** Stupid apathetic condition, with the greatest indifference. Tongue dry, with a brown streak in the middle. Confusion of thought, and when speaking forgets the word to use. Loss of consciousness, with delirium and great weakness. * Sore and bruised feeling all through the patient, which compels him to constantly change position. * If conscious, he complains of the bed being too hard. Involuntary discharges of fæces and urine.

**Ars.** Face pale, shrunken, hollow, and cadaverous, or yellowish, bluish, or leaden colored. Cold sweat on the forehead. Lips dark, dry, and cracked, with sordes on the teeth. Tongue dry, shrivelled, bluish, or black, with inability to protrude it. * Intense thirst, drinking often but little at a time. Pulse quick, weak, or irregular. Coma or low muttering delirium, and trembling of the limbs. * Extreme debility or complete prostration. * Great anguish, extreme restlessness, and fear of death. Darkish or greenish fetid stools. Typhoid abdominalis.

**Baptisia.** Face dark-red, with a besotted expression. Dull, stupefying headache, with confusion of ideas. Head feels as if scattered around, and the patient tosses about the bed to get the pieces together. Stupid and delirious. Tongue coated brown, dry, particularly in the centre. Sordes on the teeth; very offensive breath. Very fetid and exhausting diarrhœa. * The sweat, urine, and stools are all extremely fetid.

**Bell.** Face flushed and bloated, with red, sparkling eyes and dilated pupils. Throbbing headache, with violent pulsation of the carotids. * Intolerance of noise or light. Delirium, with a wild look; *he wishes to strike, bite, or quarrel.* * Starting, jumping during sleep, with desire to escape. * Sleepiness, but cannot sleep. Tongue dry, red, and cracked, or red on the edges and brown in the centre. Tenderness of the abdomen, aggravated by the least jar of the bed.

**Bry.** Face red, burning, and swollen. * Lips dry, brownish, and cracked. Tongue coated with a thick, white or yellowish fur; *later brown and dry. Oppressive, stupefying headache,* or pain as if the head would split, *worse from the least motion.* * Delirium day and night, with strange fancies, and desire to escape from bed and go home. Constant desire to sleep, with *sudden starting and strange dreams,* or sleeplessness, with restless tossing about. * Dryness of the mouth without thirst, or else great thirst, drinking large quantities at a time. * Cannot sit up from nausea and faintness. Great soreness in the pit of the stomach to touch. * Constipation, stools dry and hard, as if burnt.

**Calc. c.** Especially adapted to persons of a scrofulous habit. Palpitation of the heart, with tremulous pulse, anxiety, and restlessness. Despairing mood, with fear of death, tormenting all around him. * As often as the patient falls asleep, the same disagreeable feelings rouse him. Constant tickling under the sternum, causing a dry, hacking cough. After great anxiety and worriment of mind.

**Carb. v.** Mostly in the last stages of abdominal, and in all stages of putrid typhus. Face pale, sunken, hippocratic, cold. Eyes sunken, dull, without lustre, and insensible to light. Tongue dry, dark, and tremulous, or sometimes moist and sticky. Coma or sleeplessness, with muttering delirium. * Complete torpor of all the vital functions. Colliquative diarrhœa, brownish, grayish, or bloody, of a cadaverous smell and involuntary. * Great prostration, wants more air and to be fanned all the time. *Extremities cold, and covered with cold perspiration.*

**Cocc.** Deprivation of nervous strength, feeling weak and badly all over, but no place in particular. Slow to comprehend; he cannot find the right word to express himself. He talks in a muttering tone, requiring much effort to speak plainly. * Vertigo, especially when rising up in bed, with nausea, compelling him to lie down again. * Head and face hot, while the extremities are cold. Ringing in the ears.

**Colch.** Face sunken and hippocratic. Lips, teeth, and tongue covered with a thick brown coating. Intellect beclouded, though he gives correct answers to questions. Region of the stomach extremely sensitive to pressure. Diarrhœa; stools whitish, watery, offensive, and passed insensibly. * Cold surface, tongue, and breath; mottled skin and bluish nails.

**Hyos.** Brown-red, swollen face. Tongue red, brown, dry, and cracked. Lips look like scorched leather. *Furious delirium, which continues while awake.* Indistinct and muttering loquacity. * Muttering, with picking at the bed-clothes. Great restlessness, jumping out of bed, and endeavoring to escape. Eyes red and sparkling, staring, rolling about in their orbits. * Twitching and jerking of the limbs; *subsultus tendinum.* * Paralysis of sphincter ani and vesicæ.

**Ign.** Fever, with sudden flashes of heat. Pain in the front part of the head, which does not allow the patient to open the eyes. Choking sensation from the stomach to the throat, with oppression of the chest. * Sadness and sighing, with a weak, empty feeling at the pit of the stomach. *Numbness of the feet, legs, and sometimes of the whole lower limbs. *The patient is full of grief.

**Lach.** Dry, red or black tongue, cracked at the tip and bleeding; it trembles when being protruded. Lips dry, cracked, and bleeding. Vertigo when rising up in bed. *Stupor and muttering delirium.* Depression of the lower jaw. *Cannot bear anything to touch the throat, it is so sensitive. *Symptoms all worse after sleeping. Thinks he is dead, and that preparations are being made for the funeral.

**Lyco.** Earthy, yellow complexion. Tongue dry, black, and cracked, or covered with tough mucus. Sopor and delirium. Prostration, and depression of the lower jaw. Slow breathing, with open mouth. *Circumscribed redness of the cheeks. He uses wrong words when expressing an idea. Fan-like motion of the alæ nasi. *Bowels much distended, with rumbling, particularly in the left hypochondria. *Constant sensation of fulness in the stomach, extending up to the throat. *Great fear of being left alone. *Red, sand-like sediment in the urine. Indisposed to lie on the left side. He awakes from sleep very cross and irritable. *Worse from* 4 *to* 8 P. M.

**Merc.** In the early stage. The patient does not complain of anything in particular, yet feels so weak and ill all over that he is obliged to go to bed. Tongue dirty-yellow, or clean, with a bitter, foul taste. Gums swollen and ulcerated, with offensive breath. Headache, especially in the forehead and on the vertex. *Region of the stomach and liver very sensitive and painful. Dry, hot skin, or *copious perspiration.* Green-yellow stools, with tenesmus. Dark urine. *Symptoms all worse at night and in rainy weather.

**Mur. ac.** Advanced typhus; the patient is stupid, unconscious, and extremely prostrate. *Constant sliding down in bed. *Low, muttering delirium, groaning in sleep, and picking at the bed-clothes. Inability to protrude the tongue, which is very dry. Depression of the lower jaw, boring the head into the pillow, turning up the whites of the eyes, slavering. Involuntary stools and urine.

**Nitric ac.** Mostly in advanced stages of the disease. Inclination to looseness of the bowels, with green, slimy, acrid stools, accompanied by severe pain. * Hemorrhage from the bowels, and great sensitiveness of the abdomen. Extremely offensive urine. Irregular pulse, failing strength.

**Opi.** Face swollen and of a purplish color. * Extreme drowsiness and coma, with stertorous breathing. Delirious talking, with eyes wide open. Pulse full and labored, or slow and feeble. Impending paralysis of the brain. Involuntary stools, and retention of urine.

**Phos.** *Typhoid pneumonia.* When a large portion of the lungs is inflamed, with dyspnœa, a hard, dry, or loose cough, with *rust-colored* expectoration. Great depression of the mental faculties, mild delirium, and grasping at flocks. Dry lips and tongue, with *thirst for very cold drinks.* * Vomiting of what has been drunk as soon as it becomes warm in the stomach. Painless diarrhœa, discharges watery, greenish or black, decomposed blood. * Great sense of weakness and emptiness in the abdomen.

**Phos. ac.** * Complete apathy and indifference. Does not wish to talk, and answers very slowly. Tongue dry and cracked; teeth covered with sordes. Fixed look, with hollow, glassy eyes. Continual delirium or dull mutterings. Subsultus tendinum. * Great rumbling in the bowels, and painless, watery diarrhœa. Cold perspiration on the face, hands, and pit of the stomach. Pulse frequent, feeble, and intermittent.

**Puls.** In the early stage, and where there is much gastric disturbance. Febrile heat, mingled with chilliness, which comes on as soon as the patient is uncovered. * Thickly-coated tongue, with bad taste in the mouth in the morning. *Taste as of putrid meat in the mouth, with inclination to vomit.* Symptoms very changeable, feeling well one hour, and very miserable next. * Craves fresh, cool air, is worse in a warm room. *Mild, tearful persons.* Symptoms all worse towards evening.

**Rhus t.** Prostrate and stupid. Face red and swollen, with blue circle around the eyes. Lips dry, brownish or black. Tongue dry, red and smooth. Muttering delirium, or talking to himself. Stoppage of the ears and dulness of hearing. Dry, troublesome cough, with *oppression of the chest.* * Severe pains in the limbs, worse during rest. Diarrhœa, with profuse, watery, sanguineous, or jelly-like evacuations. * Involuntary stools, with great exhaustion. * Worse at night, particularly after midnight.

**Stram.** Loss of consciousness, with involuntary motions of the limbs and body. Earnest and ceaseless *talking.* Constant and repeated *jerking of the head up from the pillow,* and then letting it fall back again. * Loquacious delirium, with a desire to escape out of bed. Tongue yellowish-brown, and dry on the centre. Lips sore and cracked, and sordes on the teeth. * No desire for water, although the mouth is very dry. * Blackish diarrhœa, smelling like carrion. Loss of sight, hearing, and speech. Copious, involuntary discharge of urine.

**Sulph.** In psoric individuals, and where well-chosen remedies do not have the desired effect. *Burning, hot distress on top of the head, with cold extremities. Dry and brownish tongue, with great thirst. Drowsiness in the daytime, with wakefulness at night. Dull of comprehension, with inability to collect his ideas. *Early morning diarrhœa; great prostration after stool. * Frequent weak, faint spells. *Talks much in his sleep;* awakens with a start.

**Tarax.** Tearing pains in the lower extremities, worse during rest. Constant muttering to himself. Violent, tearing pain in the occiput. *Great chilliness after taking anything to eat or drink. Map-like tongue.

**Tart. em.** Typhoid pneumonia, with great rattling in the chest, and dyspnœa. * Loose cough, without expectoration. * There is apparent danger of suffocation. Acute œdema of the lungs.

**Zinc.** Entire loss of consciousness; does not recognize his own relations. Delirium, with staring eyes and efforts to get out of bed. Position on the back, and sliding down in bed. Subsultus tendinum, grasping at flocks, and feeling around as if in searching for something. * Constant trembling of the hands, and coldness of the extremities. Small, intermittent pulse. * Impending paralysis of the brain.

---

## WORM AFFECTIONS.

**Therapeutics.** Special indications.

**Acon.** When there is much febrile disturbance. The region around the umbilicus is hard, and the whole abdomen distended. Frequent ineffectual straining at stool, or nothing but slime is passed. Itching of the anus, worse at night, with restlessness. * Much fear and anxiety, the child is even afraid to go to bed.

**Bell.** Flushed face and red eyes. * Violent starting and jumping during sleep. Involuntary discharge of fæces and urine. Grating of the teeth, moaning, and uneasy sleep.

**Calc. c.** Headache, dark rings around the eyes. Pale, bloated face, and distention of the abdomen. Pain around the navel. Itching of the anus, particularly in the evening. Scrofulous persons.

**China.** If the patient has had much diarrhœa, or taken much aperient medicine. The child frequently passes worms, picks its nose much, and the belly is distended. Painless diarrhœa of undigested stools. Pain in the abdomen, worse at night, after eating.

**Cina.** * Constant boring at the nose. Frequent swallowing, as if to get something down. Restless sleep, with rolling of the eyes. Short, hacking cough, particularly at night. Abdomen hard and distended, with frequent pain in the umbilical region. * The urine turns milky after standing a short time.

**Lyc.** Earthy, yellow complexion, with blue circles around the eyes. Much flatulent distention in the stomach and bowels. Sensation as of something crawling and moving in the abdomen. *Ascarides*, with much itching about the anus. * Red, sandy sediment in the urine. Constipation of hard stools.

**Merc.** *Ascarides*, with troublesome itching of the anus; the worms crawl out, and can be seen on the perineum. Continual greediness for eating, yet grows weaker withal. Offensive breath.

**Santonine.** Many practitioners prefer this preparation to **Cina.** The symptoms indicating its use are the same as enumerated under Cina.

**Spig.** Sensation of a worm rising in the throat. Nausea every morning before breakfast, better after eating. Vomiting, with sour eructations from the stomach. Very pale face, and a yellow margin around the eyes. * Violent palpitation of the heart.

**Stann.** Discharge of mucus from the bowels mingled with ascarides. Soreness and smarting at the anus. *Frequent spells of pain in the abdomen, during which the child wishes to lean against something hard for relief.

**Sulph.** Frequent passage of lumbricoides, ascarides, and tænia. Creeping and biting in the rectum. * Gets very hungry about 11 A. M. * Frequent weak, faint spells through the day. Rawness and excoriation of the anus much of the time. Pustular eruptions on the skin.

---

## YELLOW FEVER.

**Therapeutics.** Special indications.

**Acon.** Mostly in the first stage, when there is burning heat and dry skin; full, hard, and rapid pulse. Agonized tossing about, violent thirst, red face, shortness of breath, and great nervous excitability. Delirium at night. *Headache as if everything would press out of the forehead, with vertigo on rising. Eyes injected and sensitive to light. Vomiting of mucus and bile.

**Arg. nit.** Suitable in the second stage, when there is vomiting of a brownish mass, mixed with coffee-ground-like flakes. Dizziness and much confusion in the head. Time seems to pass *very slowly.* *Green, fetid stools, passing off with much flatulence.

**Ars.** Face yellowish or livid, with distorted features and death-like countenance. Nose pointed, eyes sunken and surrounded by dark margins. Dull, throbbing or stunning pains in the head. Burning, or sharp and darting pain in the epigastrium, or in the region of the liver. Limbs feel stiff and useless. Frequent stools, with tenesmus, or painless and involuntary. * Violent vomiting immediately after eating or drinking, and of a brown and black substance. * Burning in the stomach, with great thirst, drinking little and often. *Rapid prostration.* * Extreme restlessness and fear of death.

**Bell.** In the early stage. Glowing redness of the face, with red sparkling eyes or fixed look. Throbbing headache, with visible pulsations of the carotids. * Furious delirium, wishes to strike, bite, or quarrel. Tongue coated white, yellowish, or brown. Painful heaviness and cramp-like pains in the back, loins, and legs. Cramp-like and contractive pains in the stomach. Vertigo, with vanishing of sight, stupefaction, and debility. Symptoms all worse 3 P. M.

**Bry.** Mostly in the second stage. Headache as if it would split open, aggravated by motion, opening the eyes, or stooping. Eyes red, or dull and glassy, or sparkling and filled with tears. Tongue coated white or yellow, with dry, parched, and cracked lips. * Sitting up in bed causes nausea and faintness. Food is thrown up immediately after eating. * Patient wants to keep perfectly quiet. Exceedingly irritable. Everything tastes bitter. Stools hard and dry, as if burnt.

**Camph.** Severe and long-lasting chill at the commencement. * Great coldness of the skin, yet cannot bear to be covered. *Prostration.*

**Canth.** Complete insensibility, cramps in the abdominal muscles and legs; suppression of urine. Hemorrhage from the stomach and intestines. Cold sweat on the hands and feet. *Constant desire to urinate.

**Carb. v.** Last stage; hemorrhages, with great paleness of the face, violent headache, great heaviness in the limbs and trembling of the body. *Patient wants more air, and to be fanned all the time. * Great foulness of all the secretions.

**Crotalus.** Hemorrhages from the eyes, nose, mouth, stomach, and intestines. Tongue scarlet-red, or brown and swollen. Fetid diarrhœa.

**Ipec.** First stage, when there is vertigo, chilliness, pain in the back and limbs; uncomfortable feeling in the epigastrium. * Continual nausea, with vomiting of glairy mucus.

**Merc.** Skin yellow, red, injected; eyes sensitive to light. Paralysis of one or more limbs. Drowsy, or sleepless from nervous irritation. Dizziness, or violent pain in the head. Violent vomiting of mucus and bilious matters. Burning pain and tenderness of the stomach. Diarrhœa, with discharges of mucus, bile, or blood, with tenesmus. * Much perspiration without relief. Great weakness of memory. Aggravation at night and in damp weather.

**Nux v.** Yellow skin, pale or yellowish face, especially around the nose and mouth. Eyes injected, yellow, and watery, with dark rings around the same. Tongue slimy, or dry, cracked, and red on the edges. Burning pains in the stomach; pressure or cramp-like pains in the epigastrium. Vomiting of acid, bilious, or mucous matters. Burning pains at the neck of the bladder, with difficulty in urinating. Coldness, paralysis, and cramps in the legs. * Very irritable, and wishes to be alone. Persons of *intemperate habits.* Aggravation in the morning.

**Rhus t.** Dirty-yellow color of the body. Eyes glazed and sunken. Tongue and lips dry and brownish. Loquacious delirium, or coma with stertorous breathing. Constant moaning and shifting about. Distressing pain and burning in the stomach. * Great weakness of the lower extremities, can hardly draw them up. Difficult and painful deglutition. * Worse at night, particularly after midnight.

**Sulph.** Face pale or yellowish. Tongue dry, rough, and reddish, with white or brownish, bloody or purulent saliva. Itching and burning pain in the eyes. Vomiting of bilious, acid, bloody, or blackish matters. * Burning on top of the head. * Frequent weak, faint spells. Trembling and weakness.

**Tart.** Nausea or vomiting, with a sense of sinking at the stomach, as if he could not survive a moment. General prostration of the whole system. Profuse cold sweat, rapid and weak pulse. Drowsiness, and disposition to go to stool.

**Verat. a.** Yellowish or bluish face, cold, and covered with *cold perspiration.* Lips and tongue dry, brown, and cracked. Trembling and cramps of the feet, hands, and legs. *Violent vomiting of green or black bile, with great weakness after. Diarrhœa, stools thin, blackish, or yellow. *Intense thirst for cold drinks.* Excessive weakness. Pulse almost imperceptible. *Cramps of the limbs, with cold sweat.

THE END.

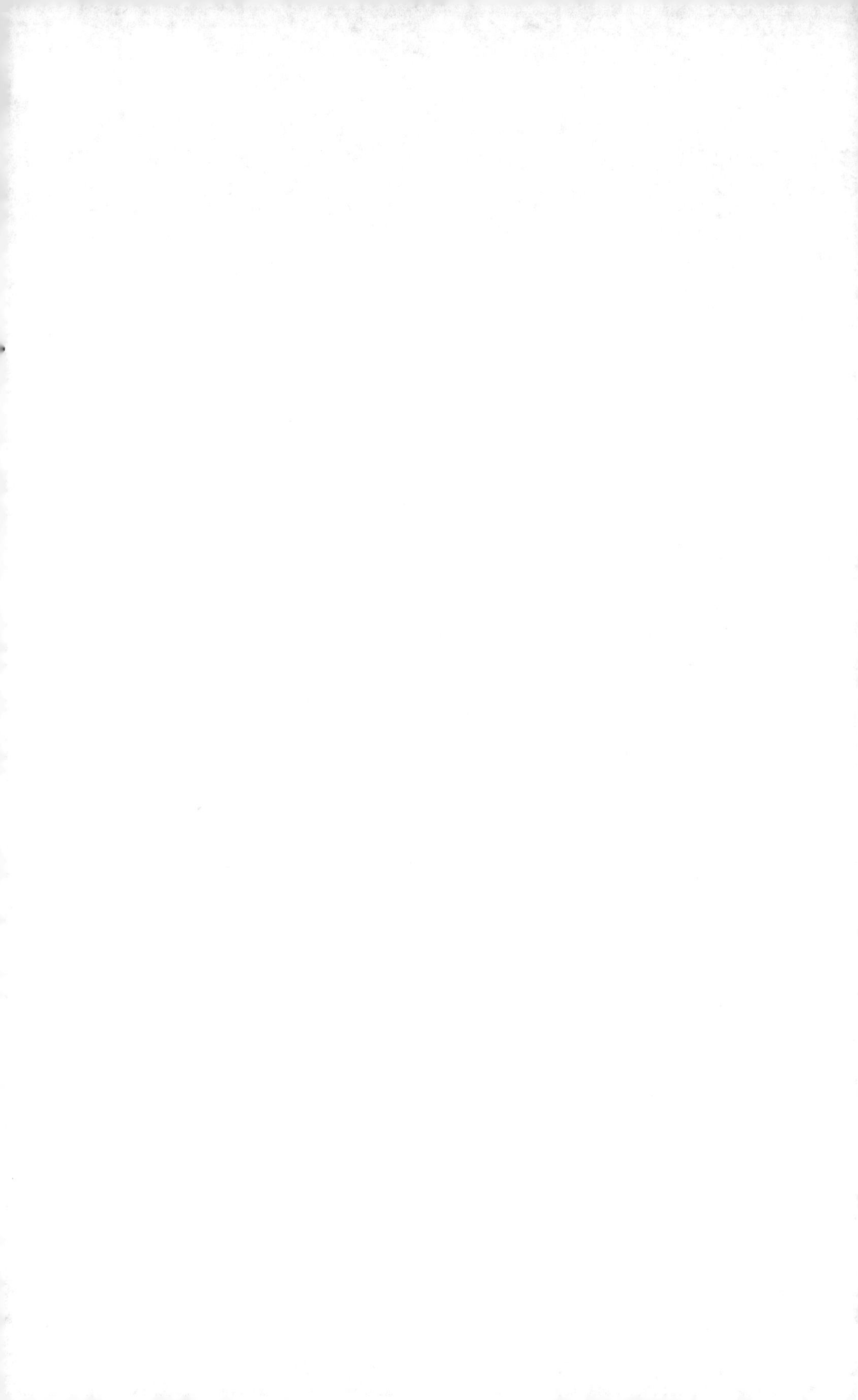

www.ingramcontent.com/pod-product-compliance
Lightning Source LLC
LaVergne TN
LVHW011232110826
845150LV00006B/1620

* 9 7 8 1 4 2 5 5 1 4 9 0 7 *